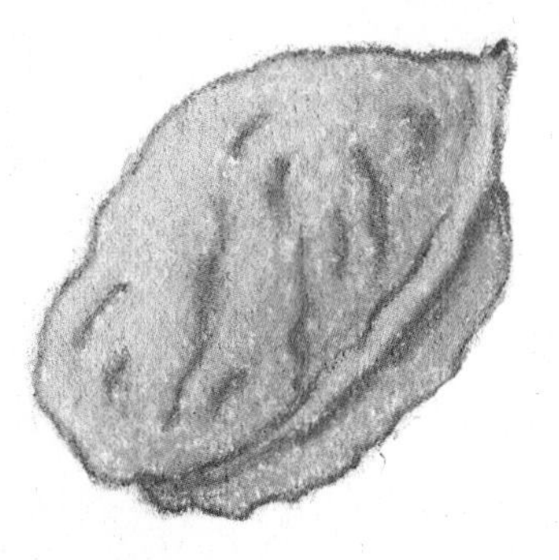

We Eat Food That's Fresh!

Written by
Angela Russ-Ayon

Illustrated by
Cathy June

Published by

OurRainbowPress
Marietta, Georgia
Printed in Atlanta, Georgia

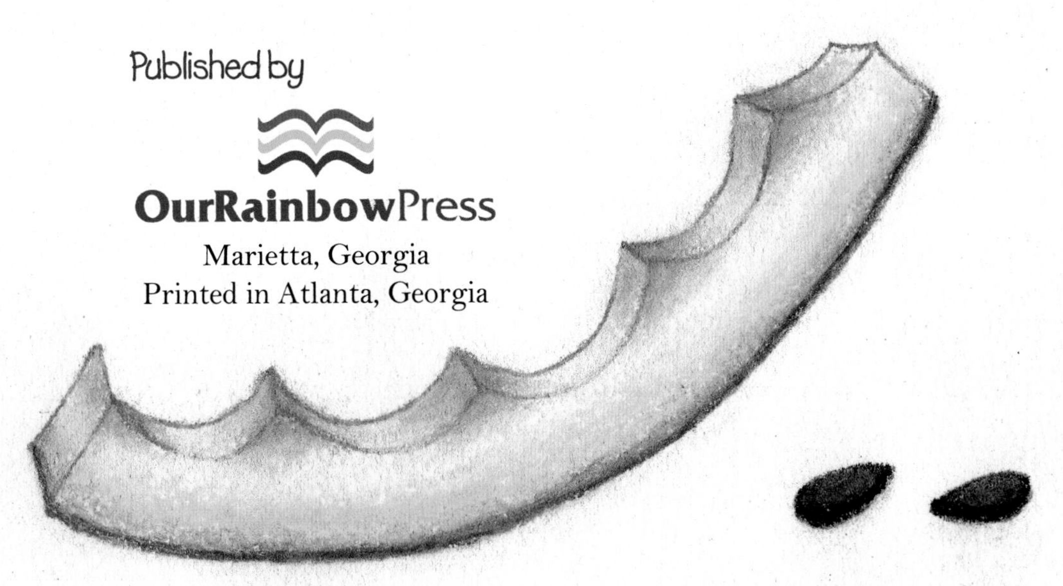

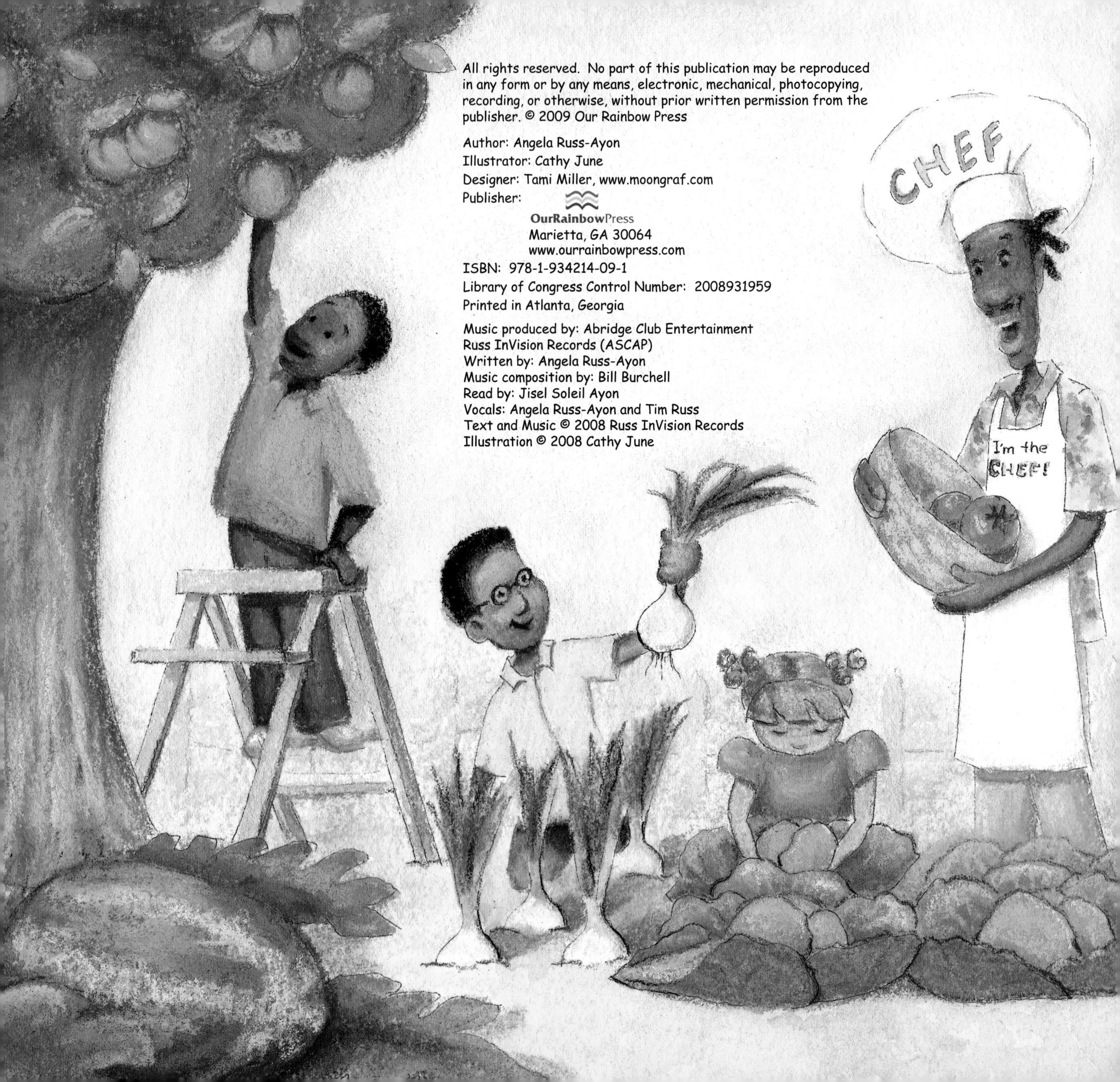

Author: Angela Russ-Ayon
Illustrator: Cathy June
Designer: Tami Miller, www.moongraf.com
Publisher:
OurRainbowPress
Marietta, GA 30064
www.ourrainbowpress.com
ISBN: 978-1-934214-09-1
Library of Congress Control Number: 2008931959
Printed in Atlanta, Georgia

Music produced by: Abridge Club Entertainment
Russ InVision Records (ASCAP)
Written by: Angela Russ-Ayon
Music composition by: Bill Burchell
Read by: Jisel Soleil Ayon
Vocals: Angela Russ-Ayon and Tim Russ

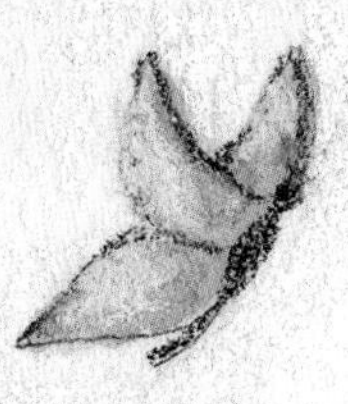

To my loving husband, Jose, for standing by me while I follow my dreams, and to my two children, Jisel and Marcos, who sing for me, play with me, and inspire me every moment of every day.

—Angela Russ-Ayon

To my husband, Mike and my family for all your support and encouragement. Bon Appétit!

— Cathy June

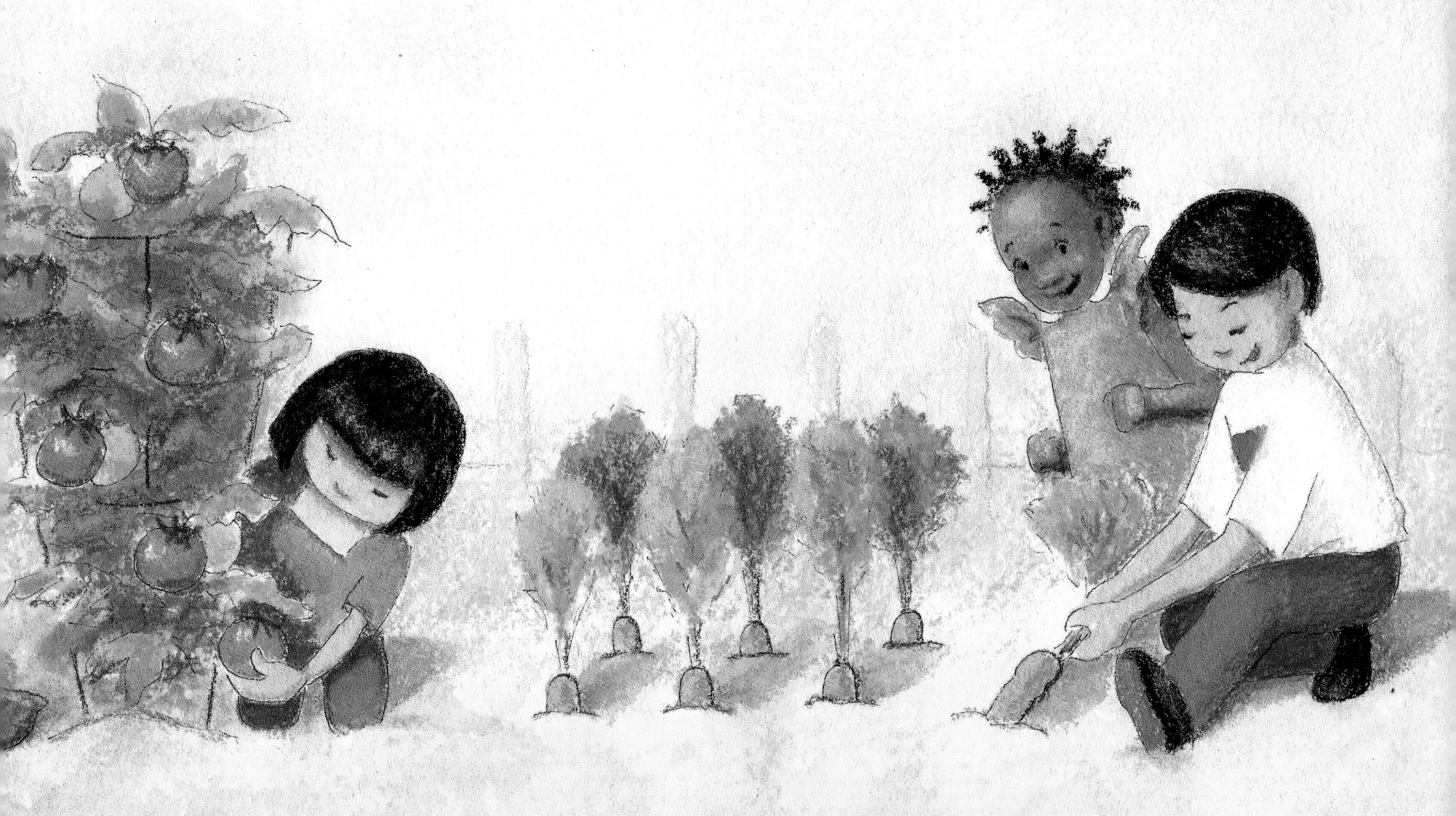

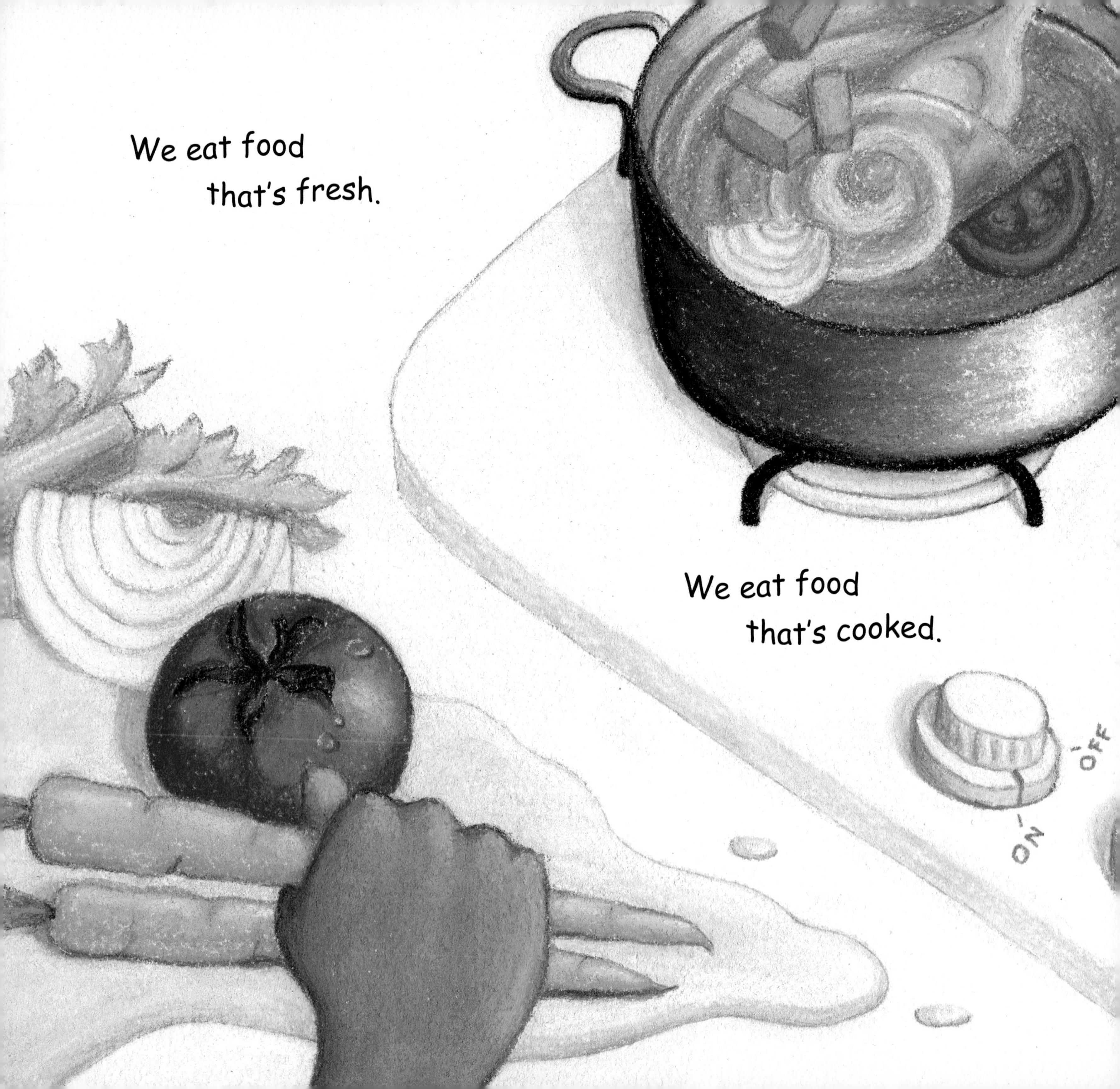

We eat food
that's fresh.

We eat food
that's cooked.

We eat food prepared
from a recipe book.

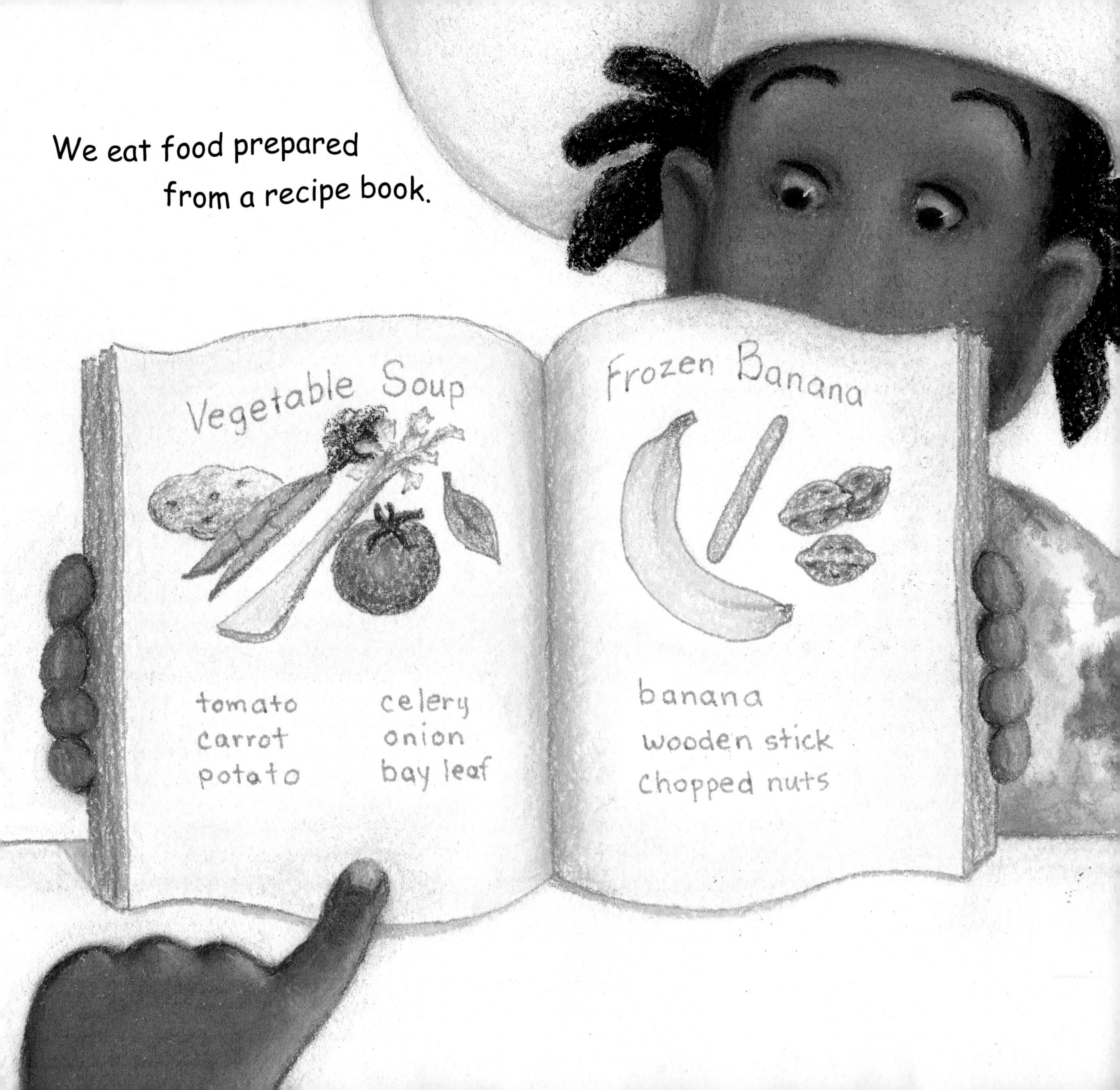

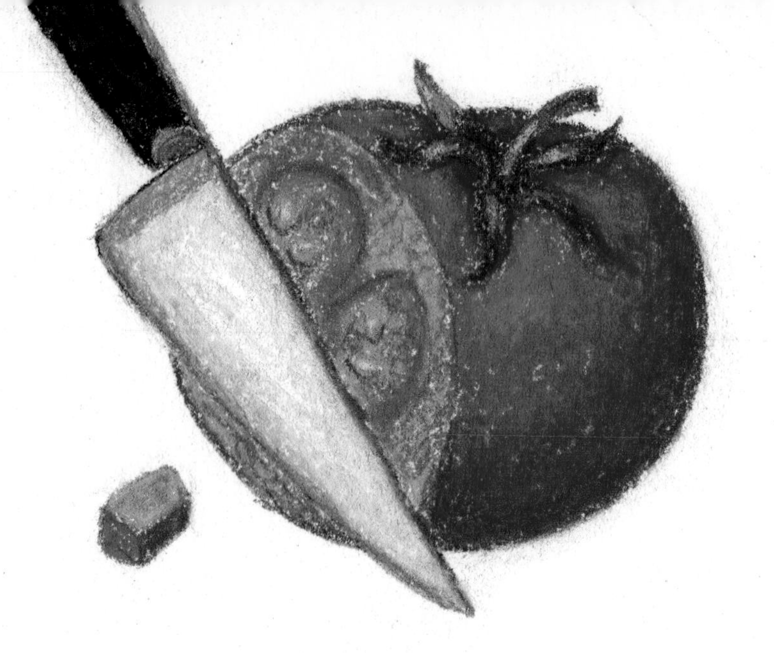

We eat food
that's chopped.

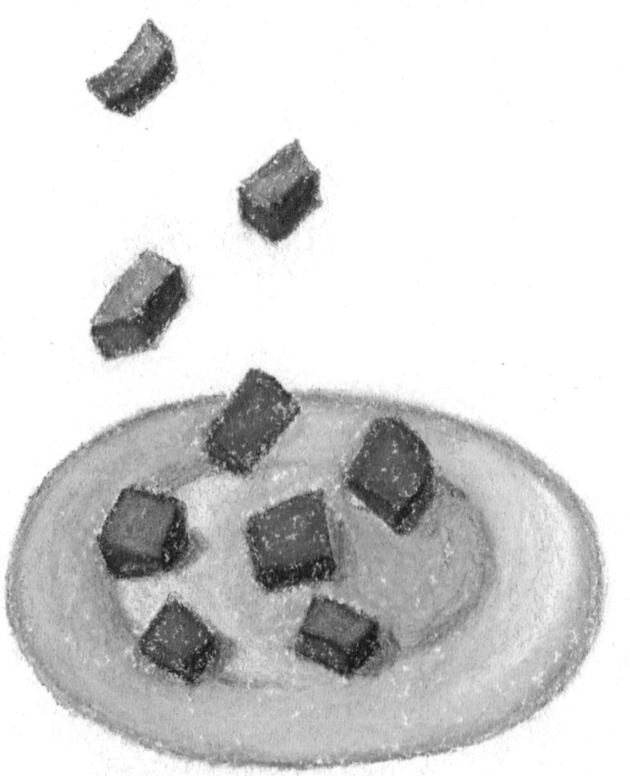

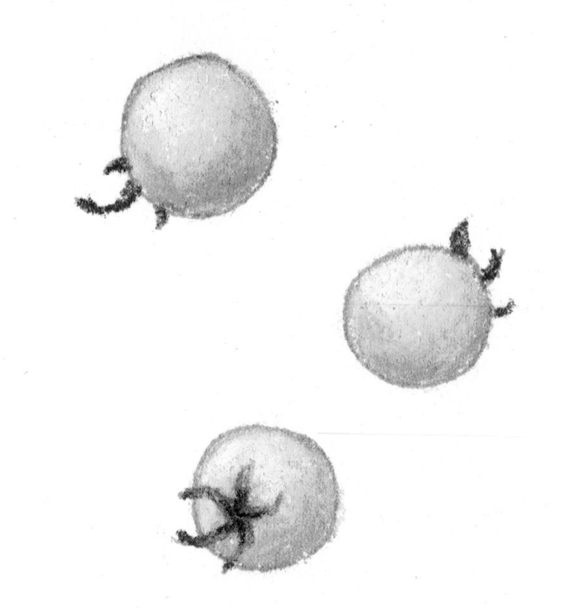

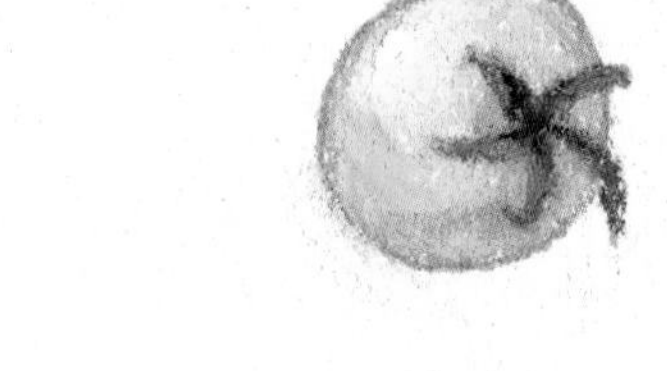

We eat food
that's not.

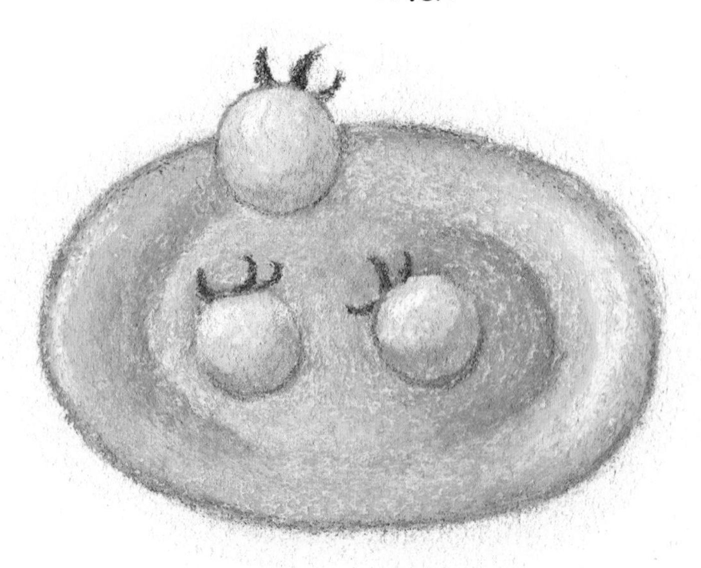

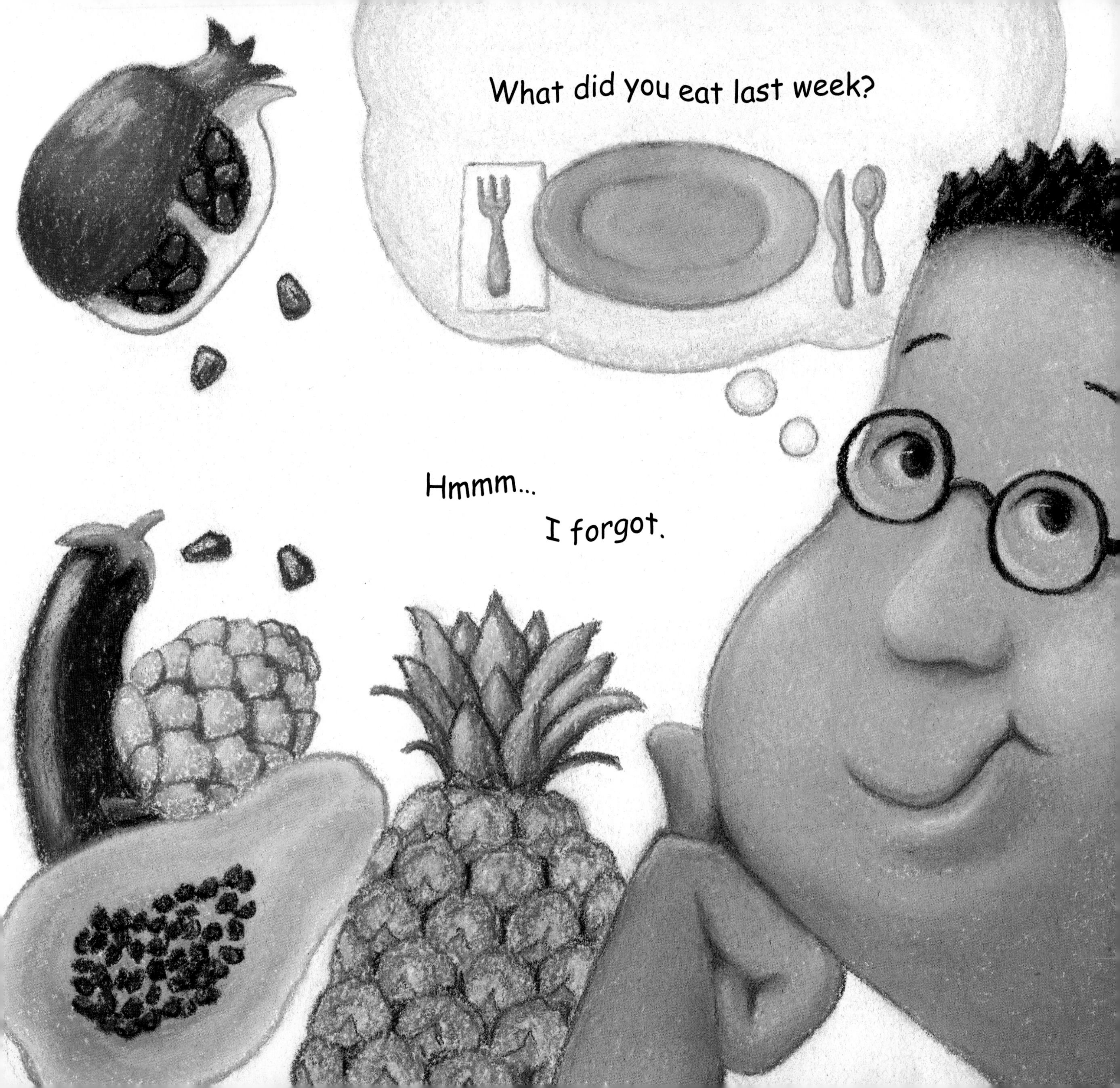
What did you eat last week?
Hmmm...
I forgot.

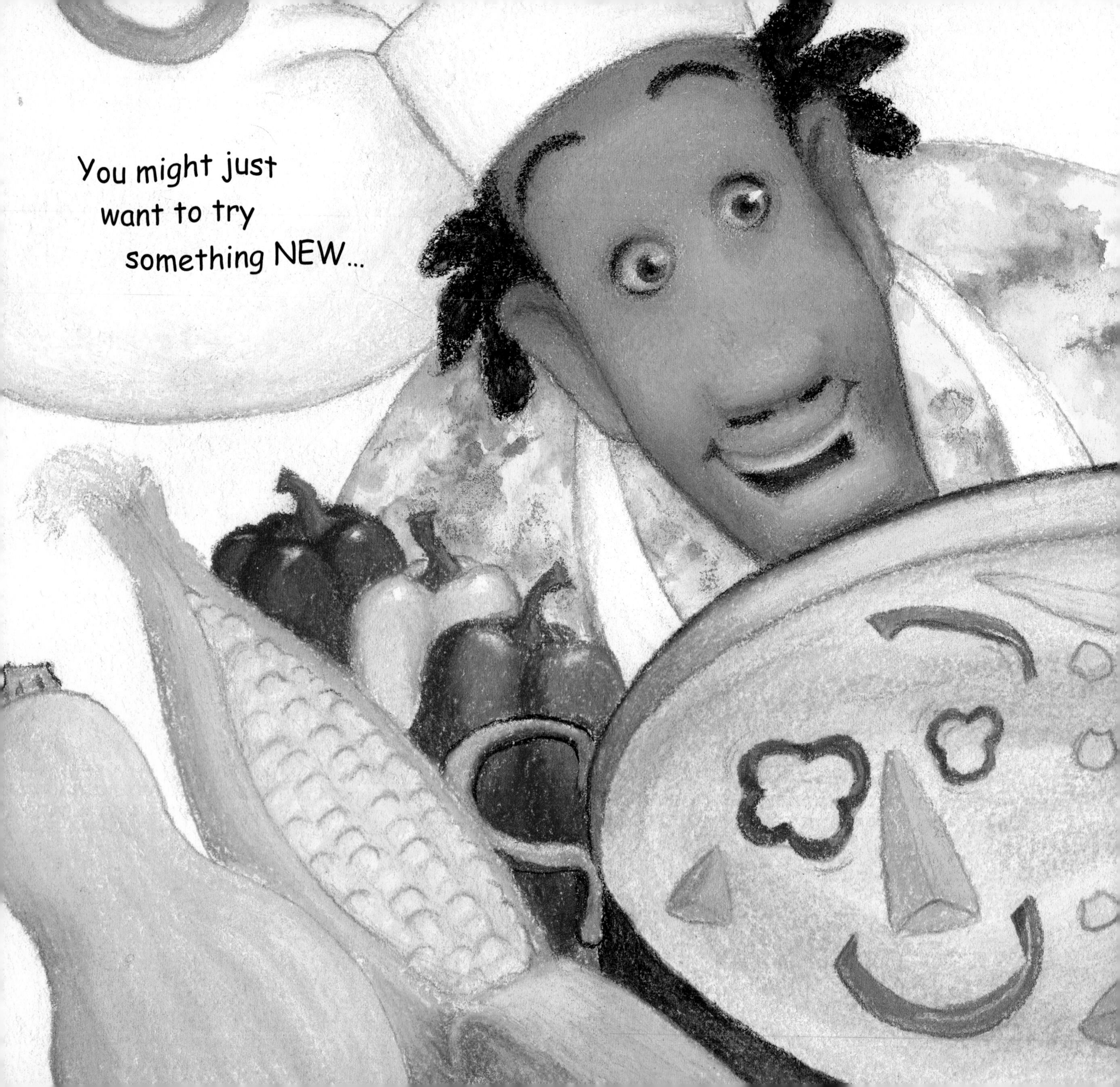
You might just
want to try
something NEW...

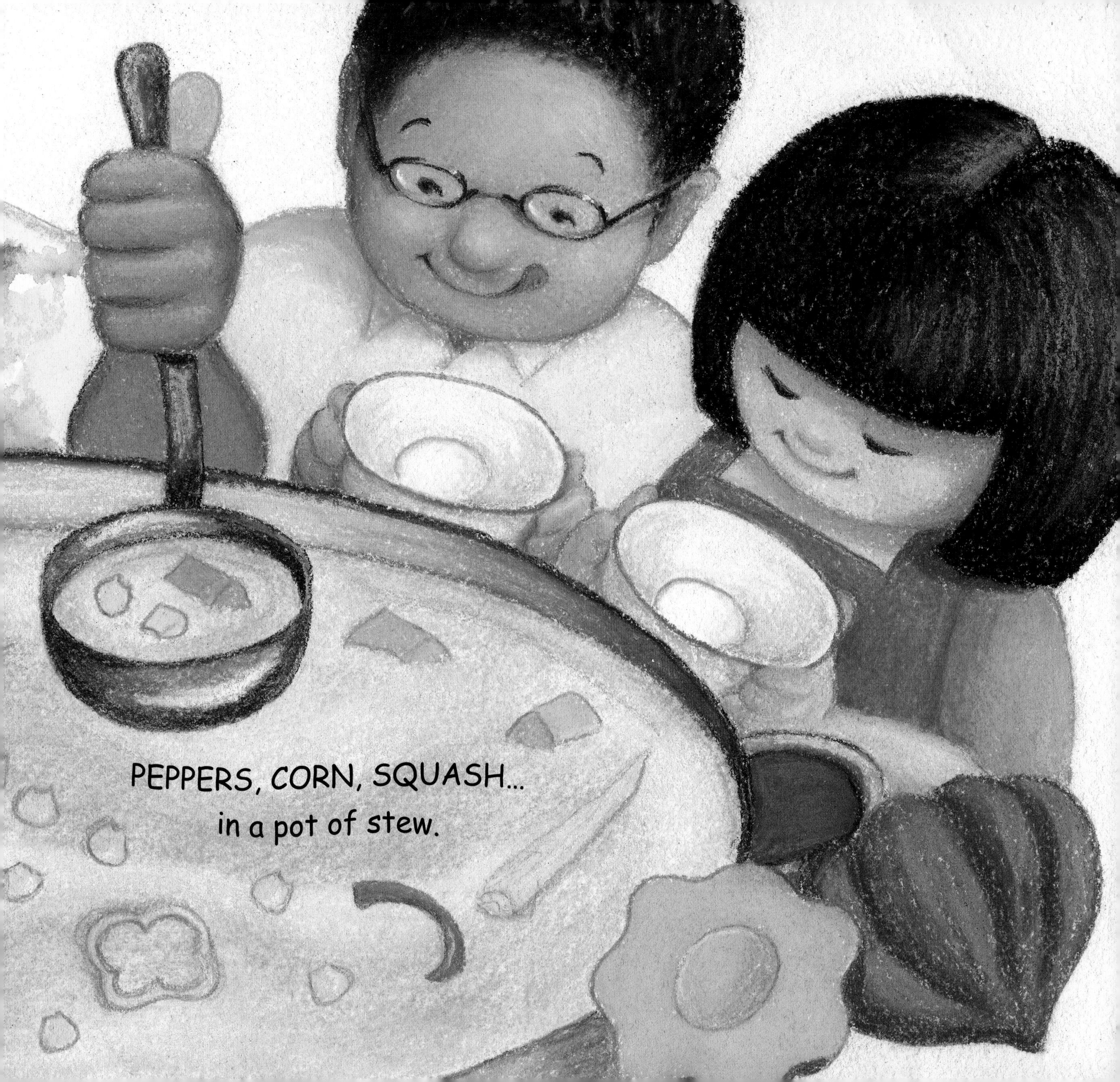

PEPPERS, CORN, SQUASH...
in a pot of stew.

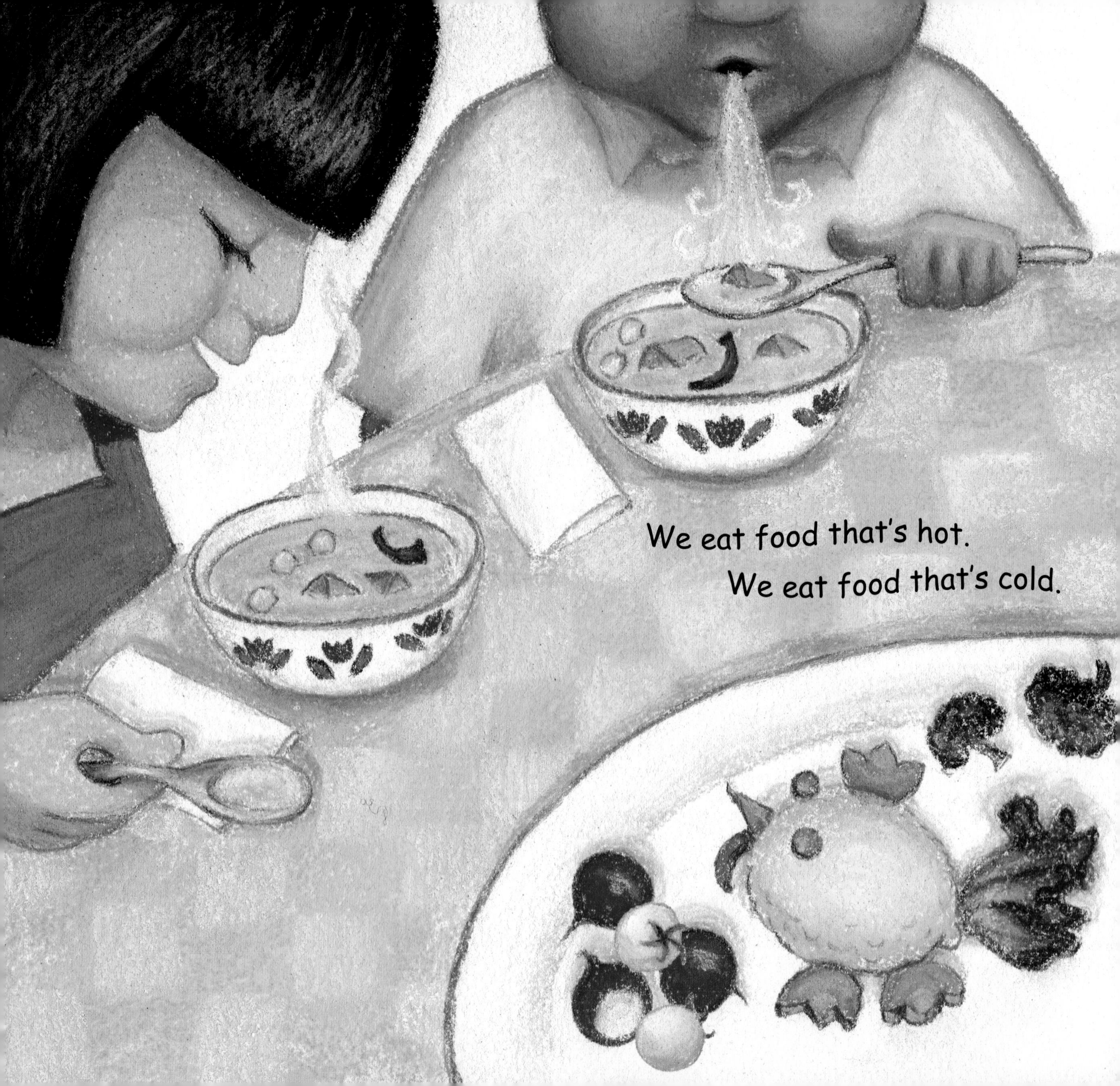

We eat food that's hot.
We eat food that's cold.

We eat food that's grown.

We eat food that's sold.

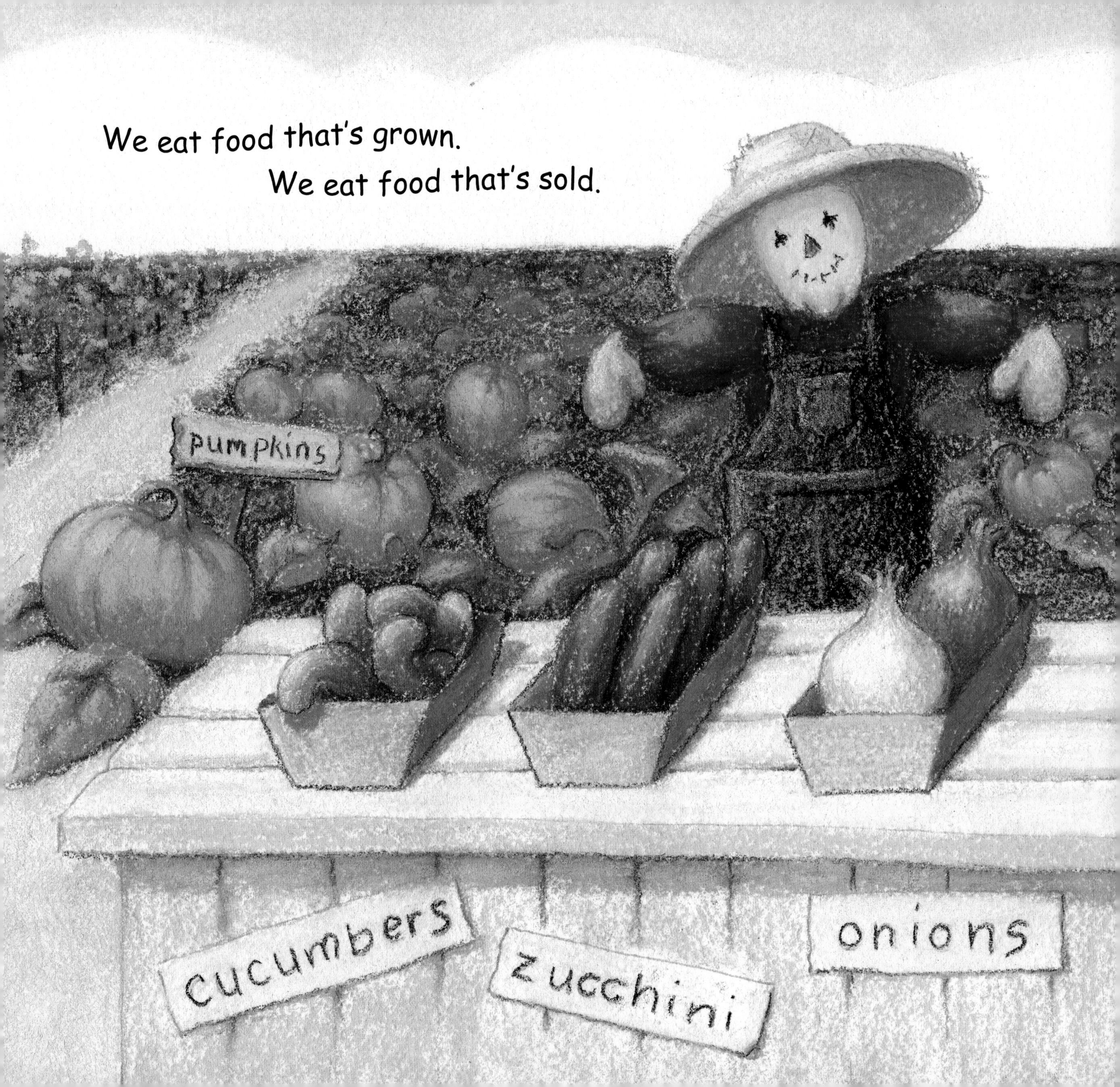

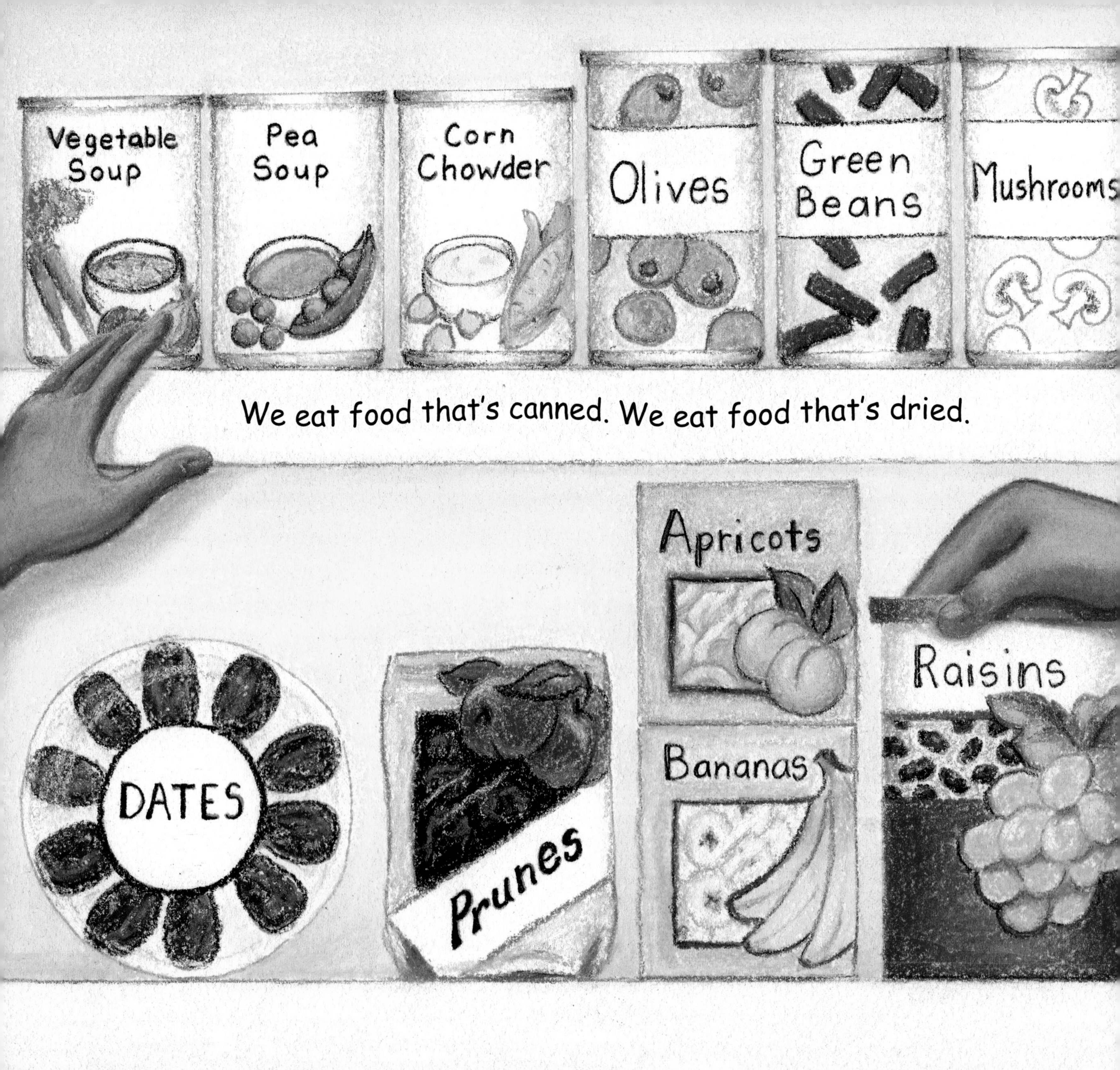

We eat food that's canned. We eat food that's dried.

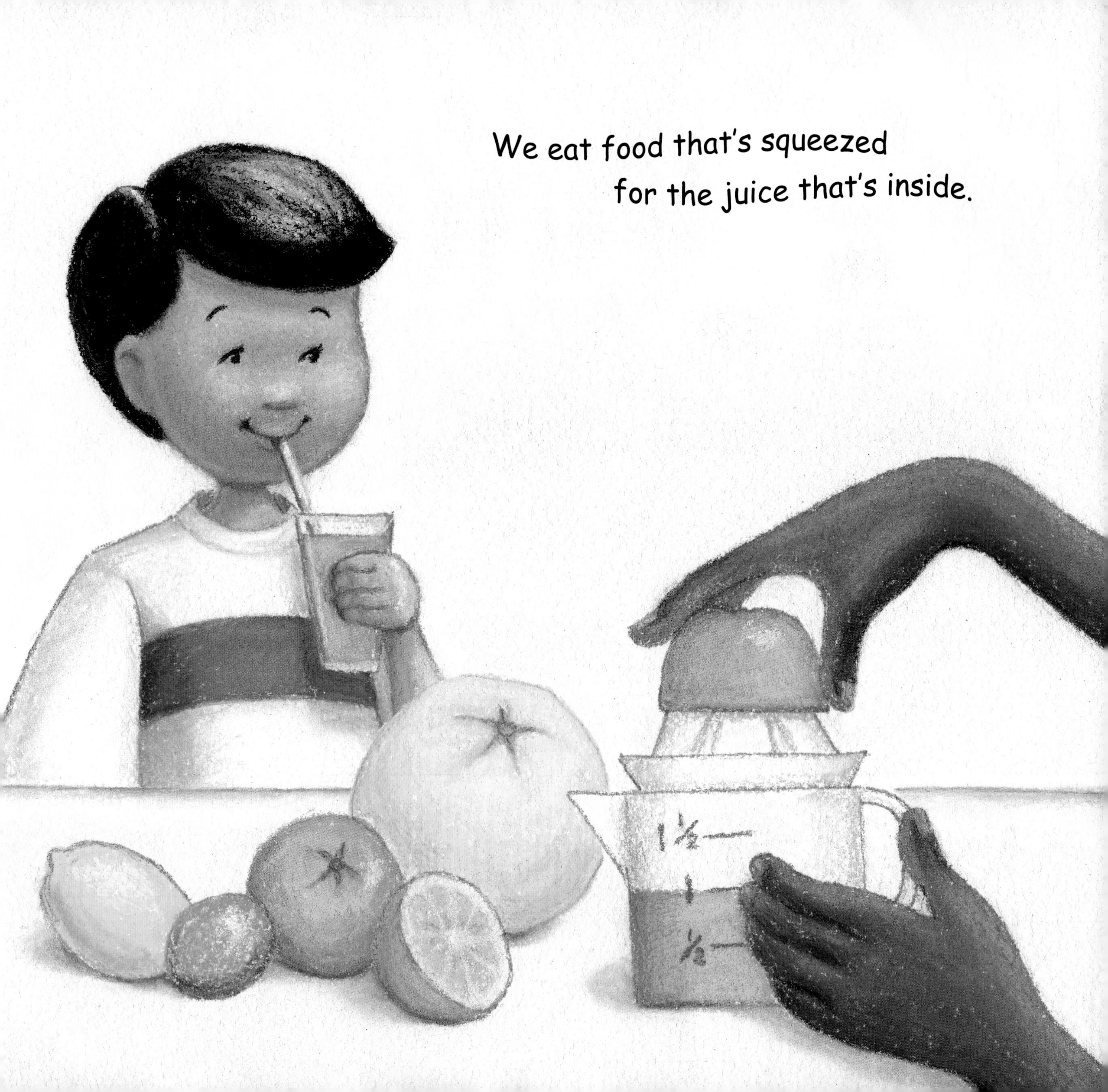

We eat food that's squeezed
for the juice that's inside.

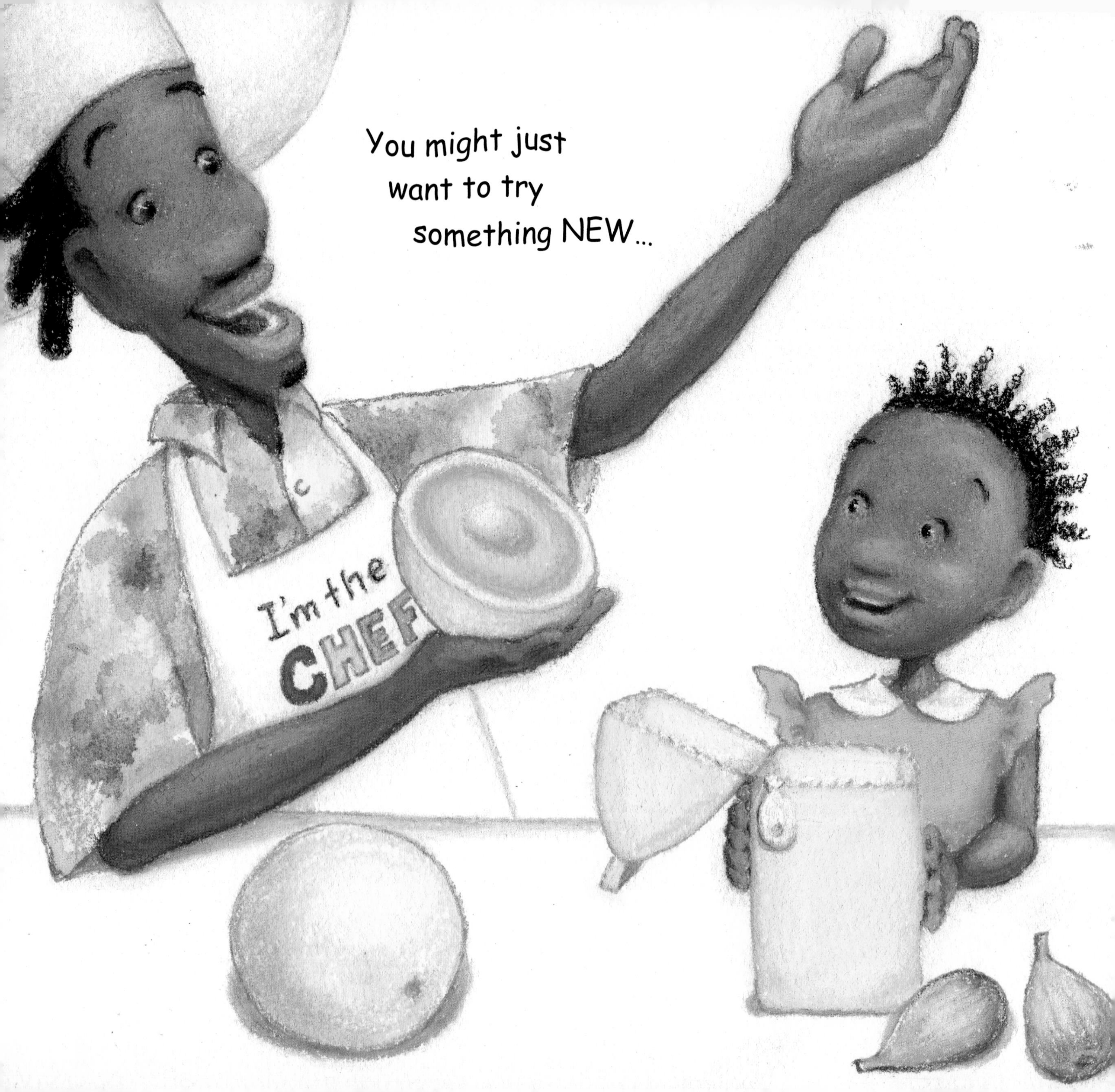

You might just
want to try
something NEW...

FIGS, DATES, KIWI, or some HONEYDEW.

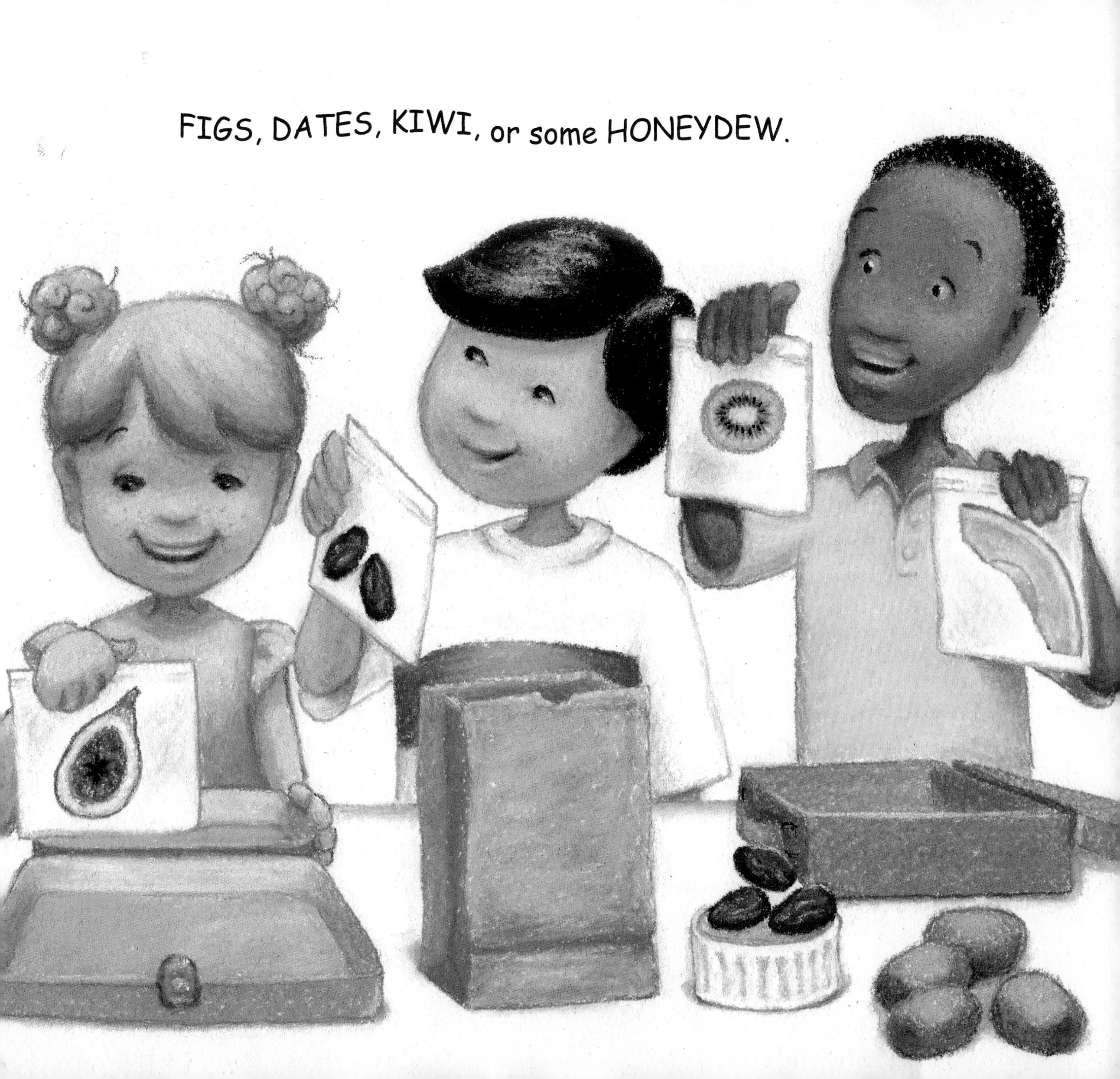

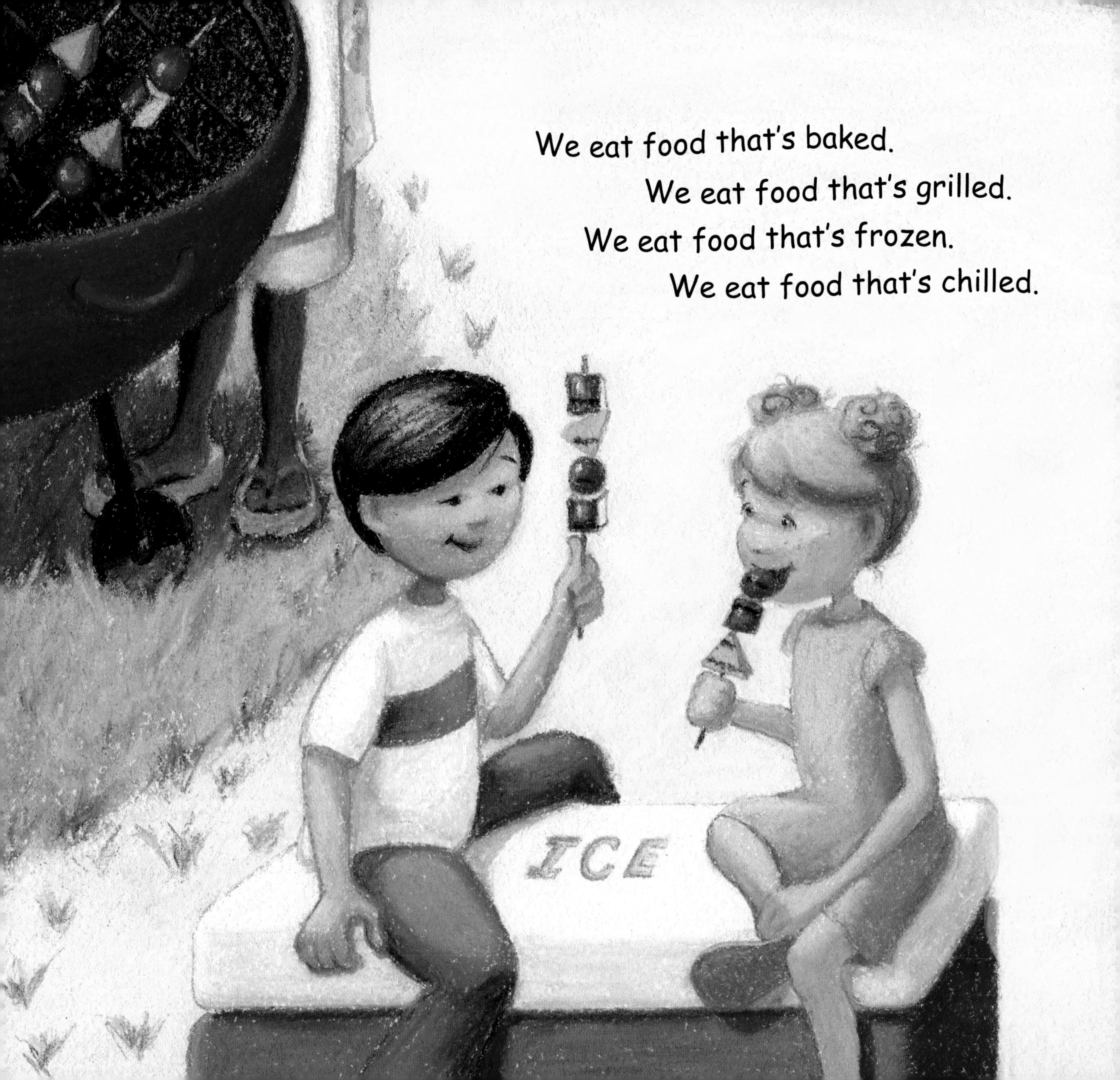

We eat food that's baked.
We eat food that's grilled.
We eat food that's frozen.
We eat food that's chilled.

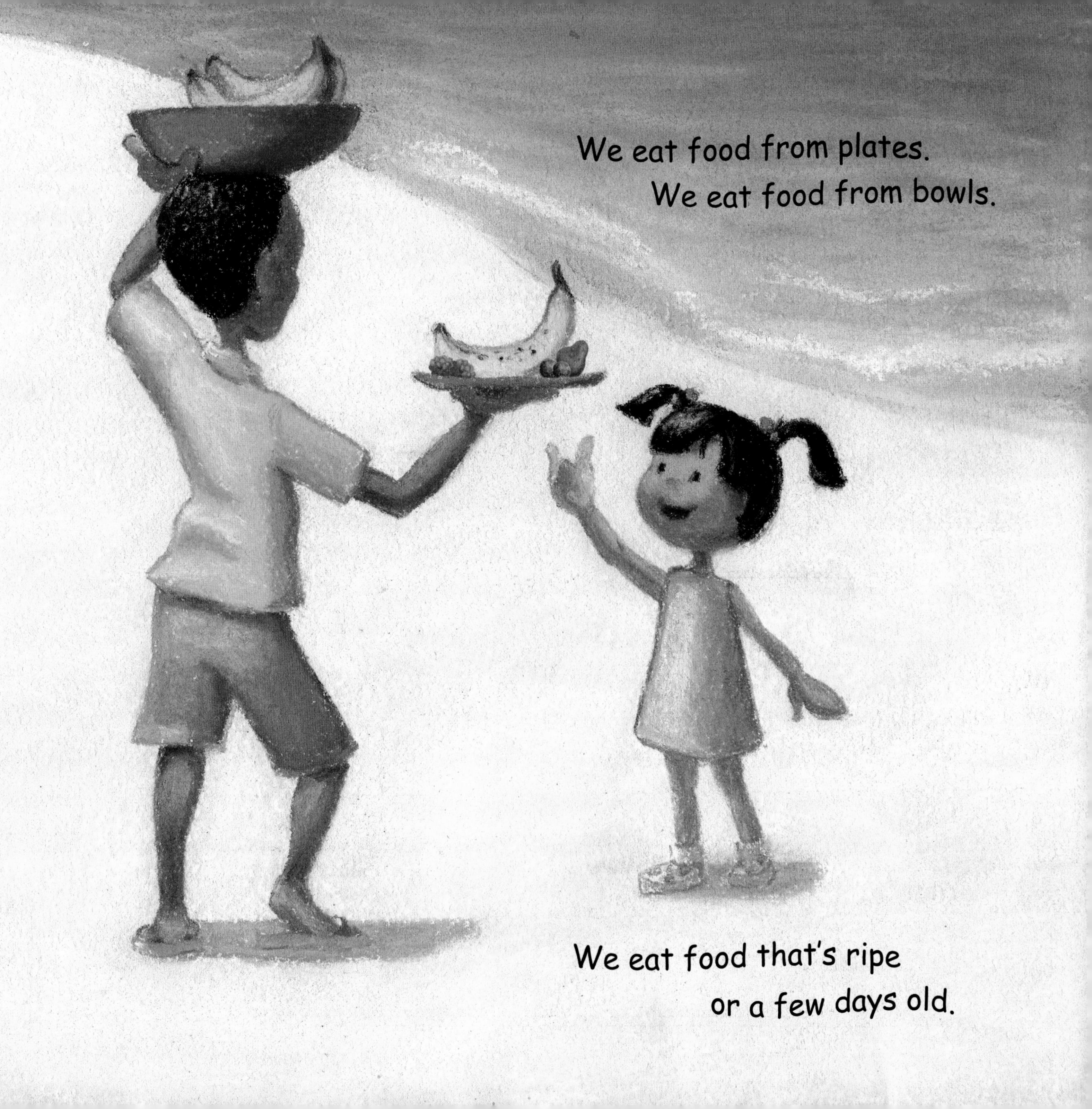

We eat food from plates.
We eat food from bowls.

We eat food that's ripe
or a few days old.

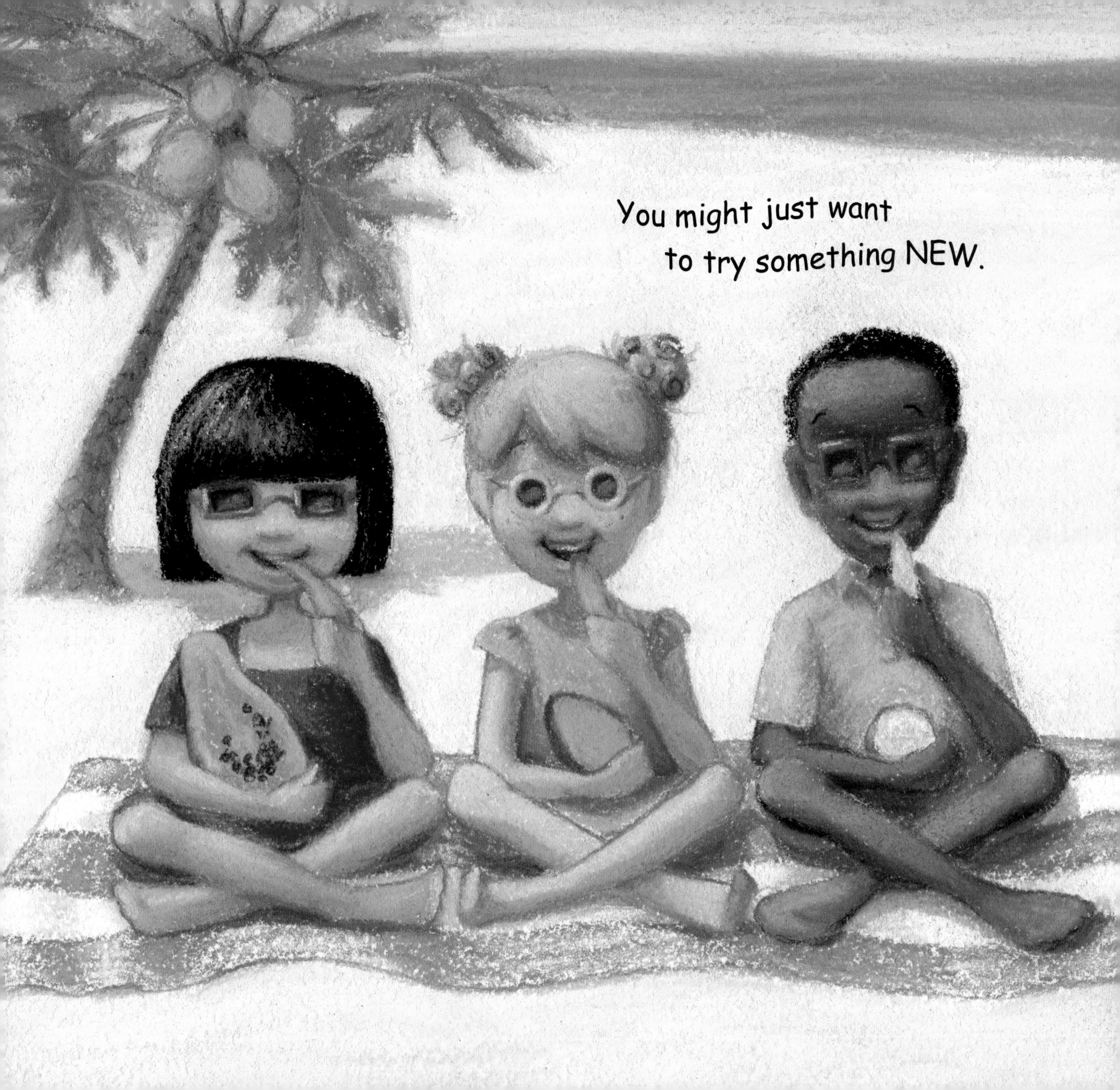

You might just want
to try something NEW.

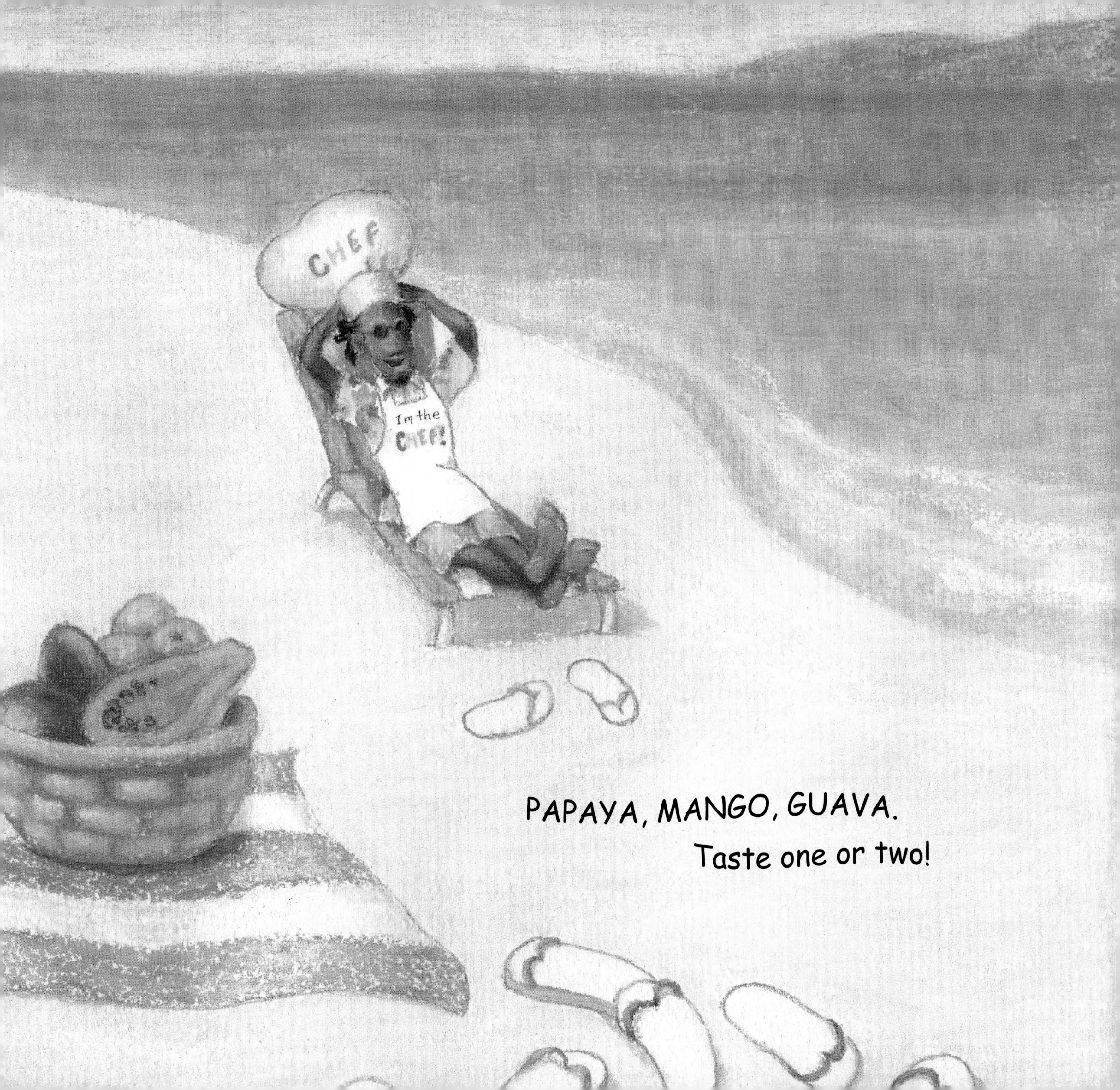

PAPAYA, MANGO, GUAVA.

Taste one or two!

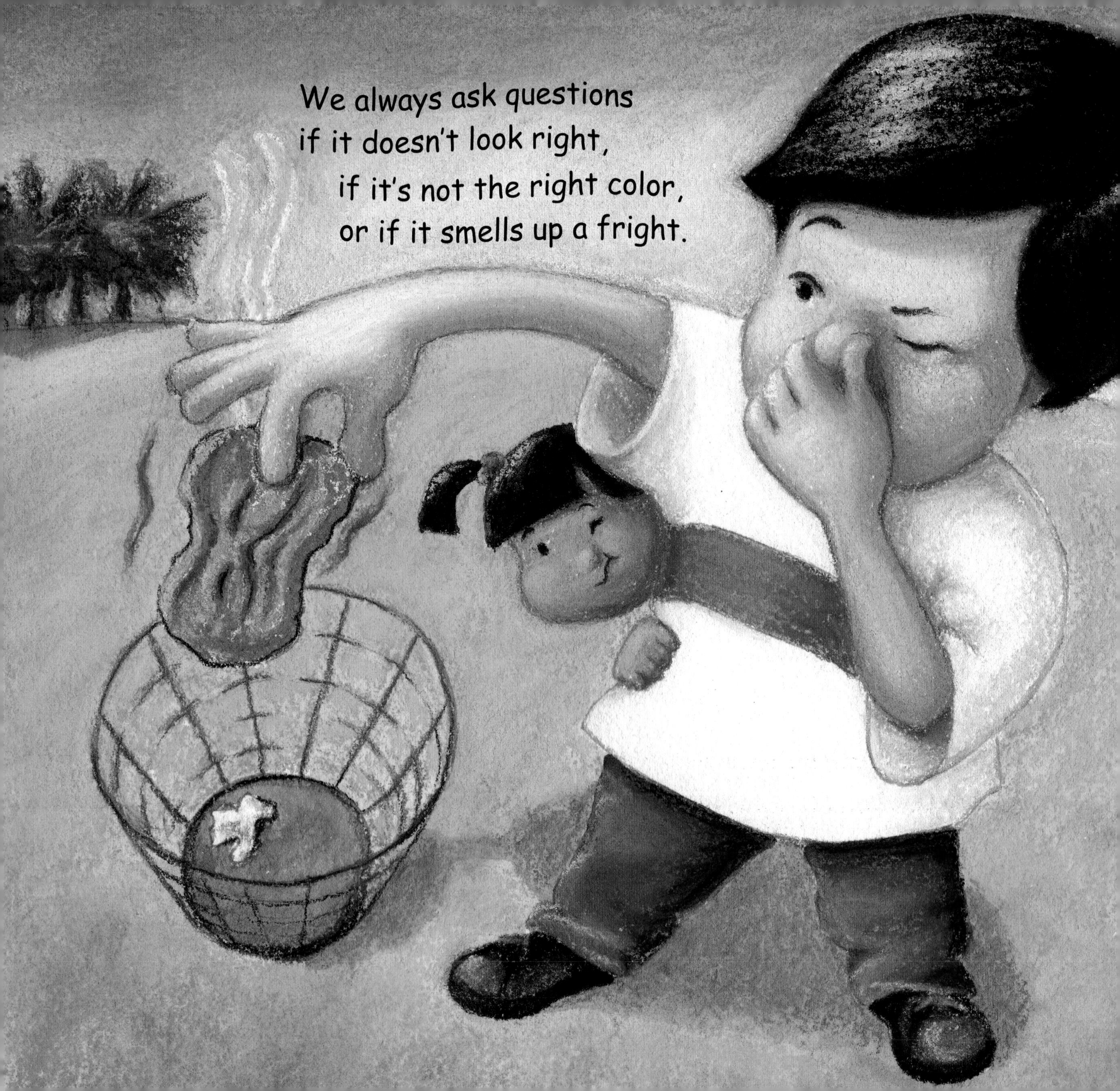

We always ask questions
if it doesn't look right,
if it's not the right color,
or if it smells up a fright.

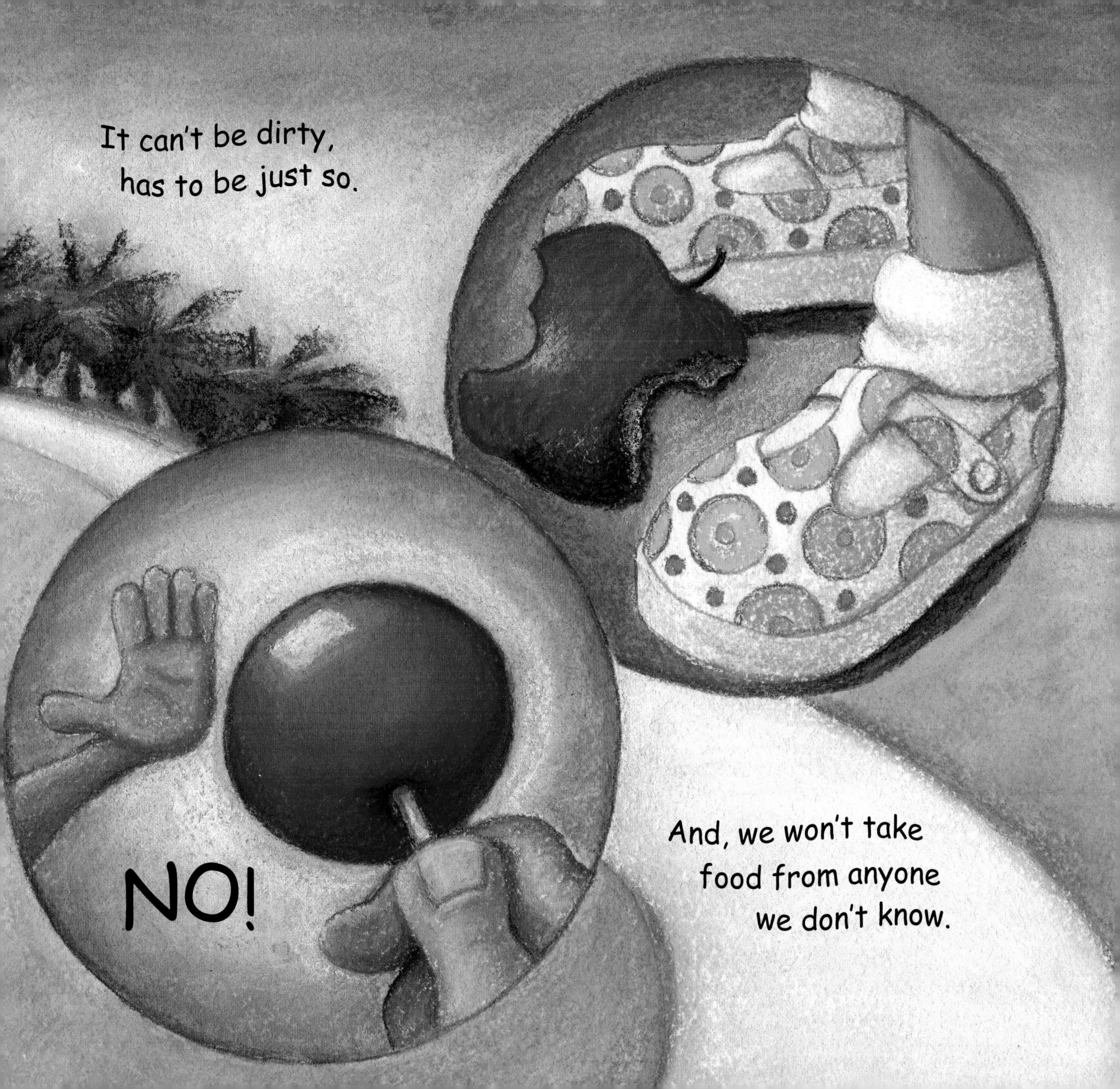
It can't be dirty,
has to be just so.
NO!
And, we won't take
food from anyone
we don't know.

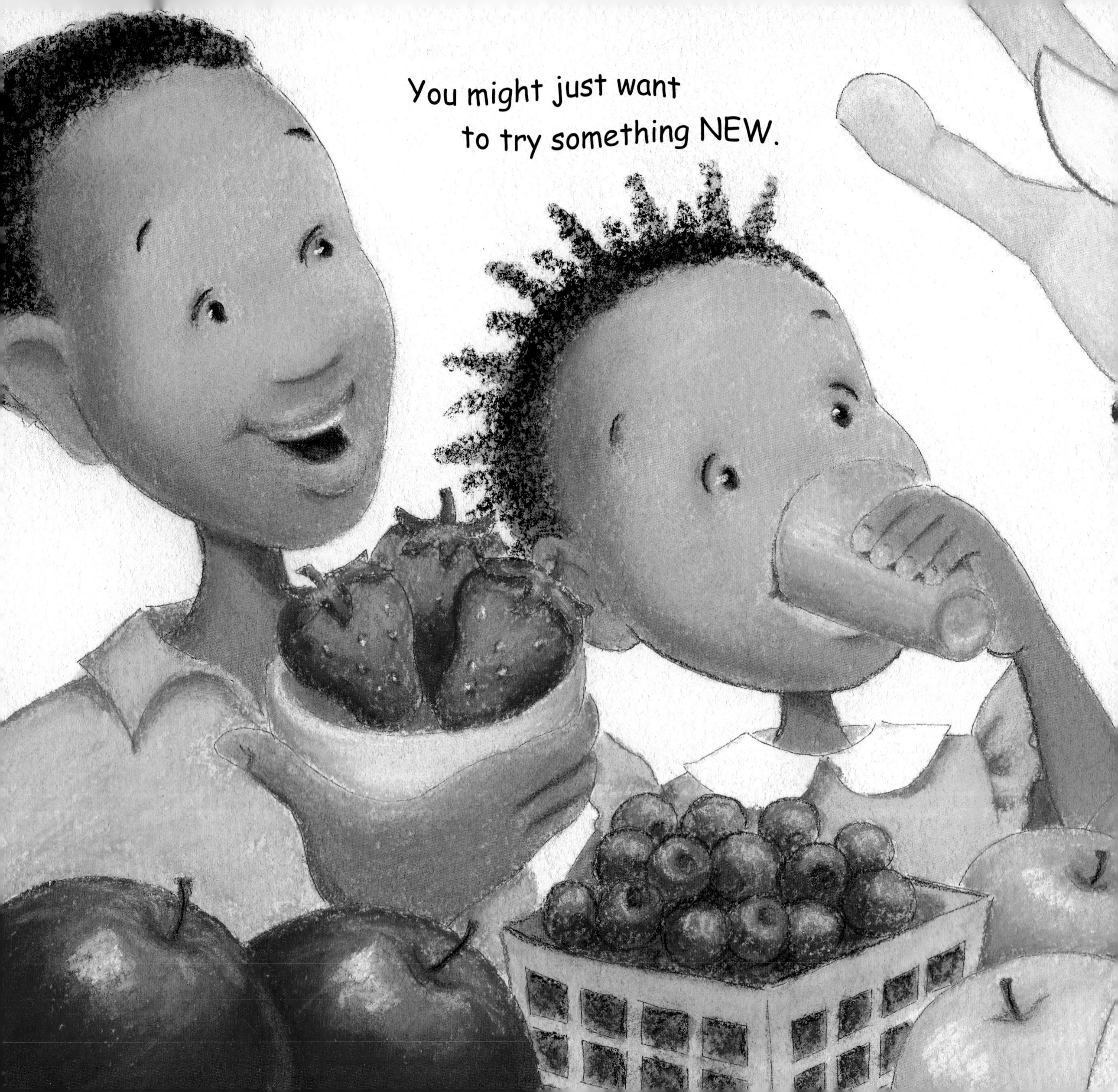

You might just want
to try something NEW.

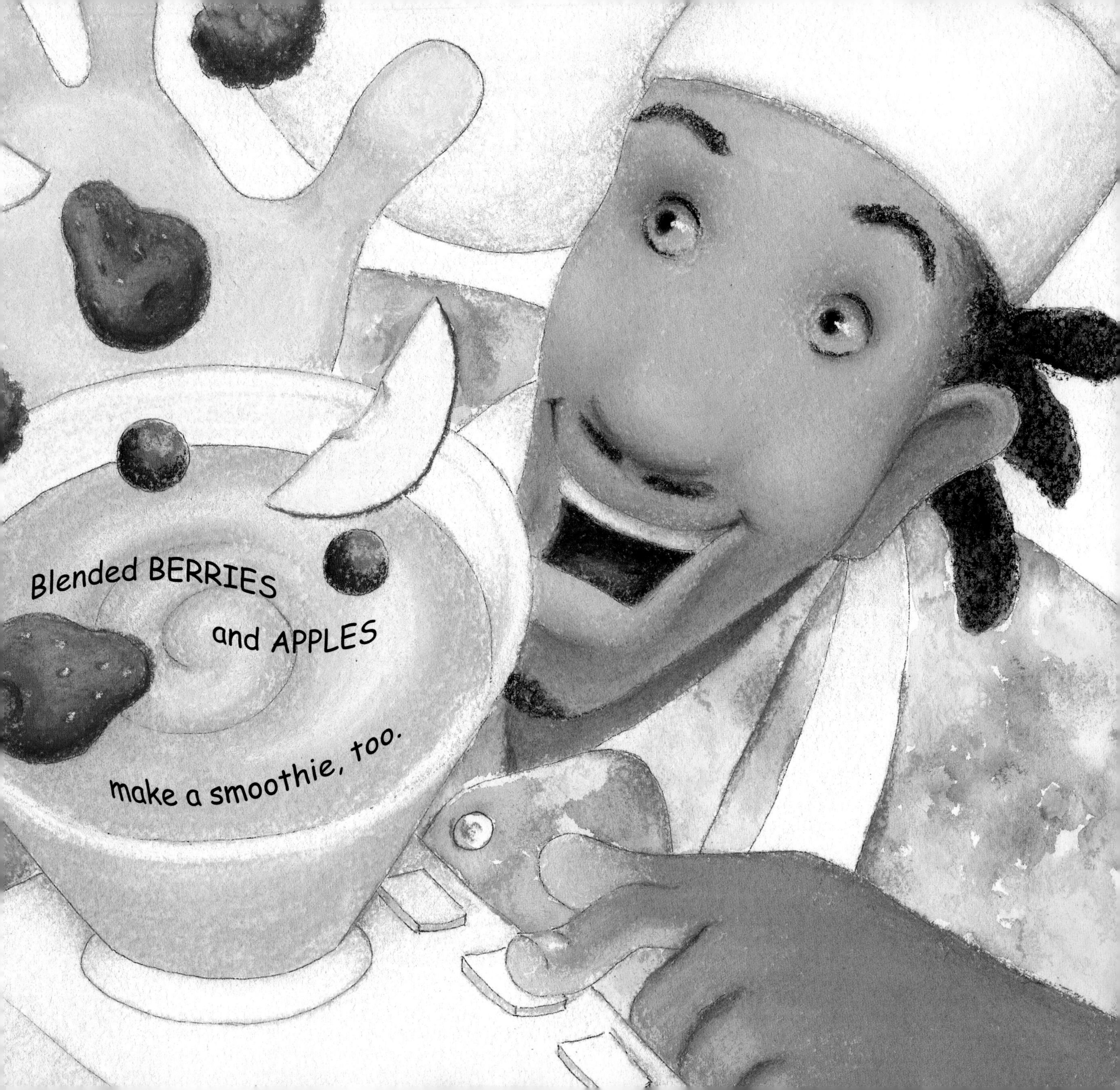
Blended BERRIES
and APPLES
make a smoothie, too.

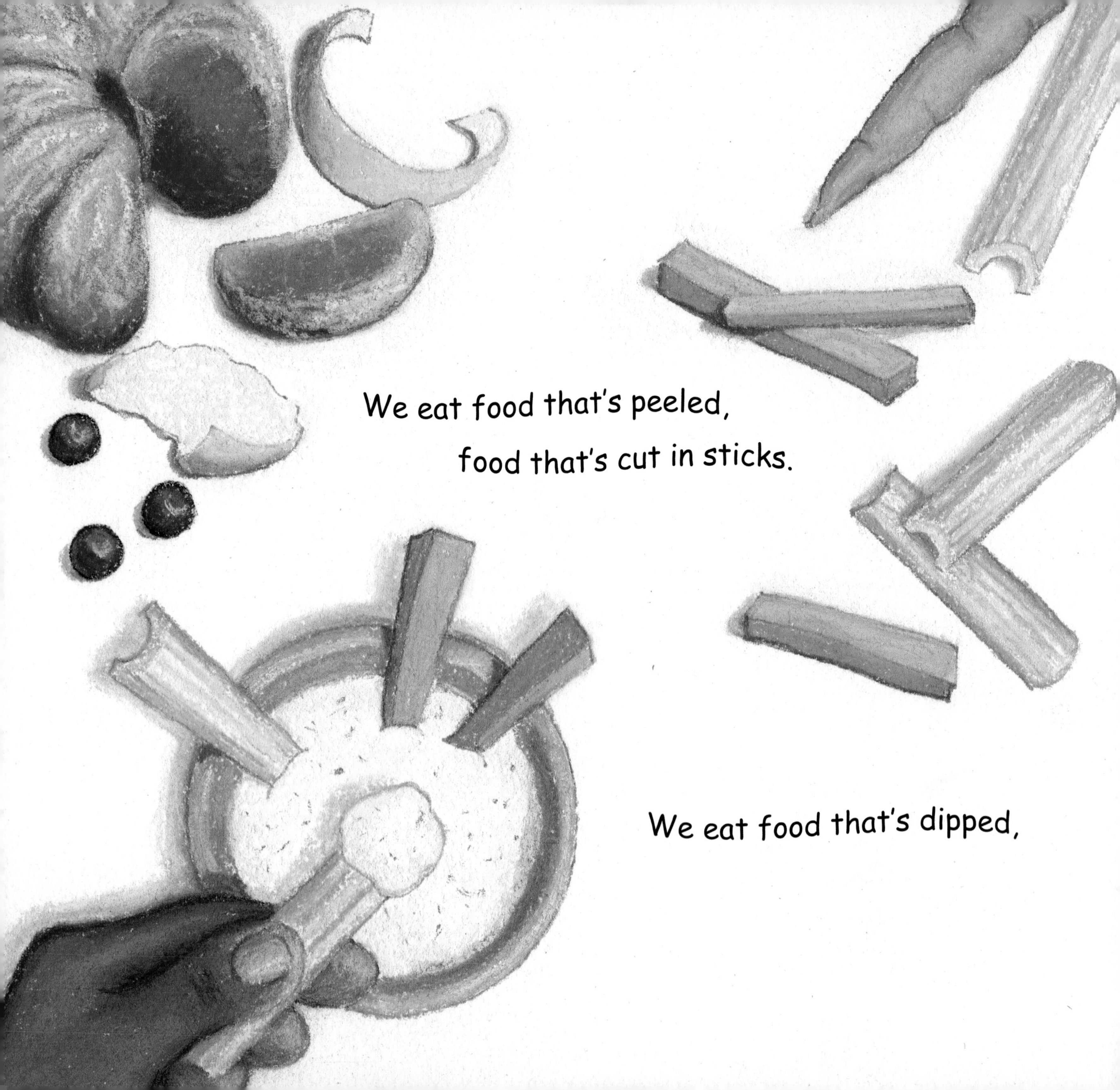

We eat food that's peeled,

food that's cut in sticks.

We eat food that's dipped,

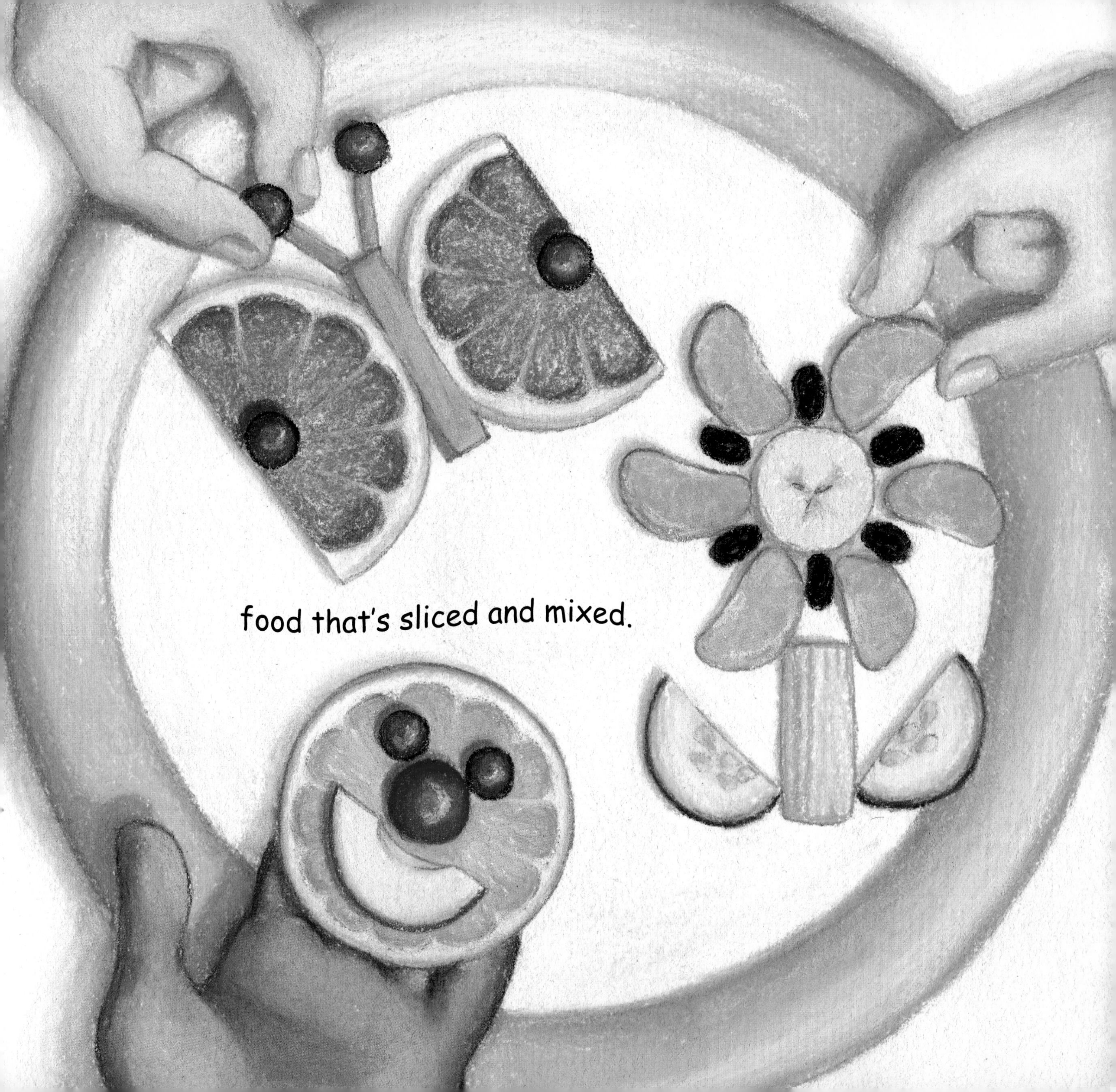

food that's sliced and mixed.

We eat food stir-fried.
We eat food that's creamed.

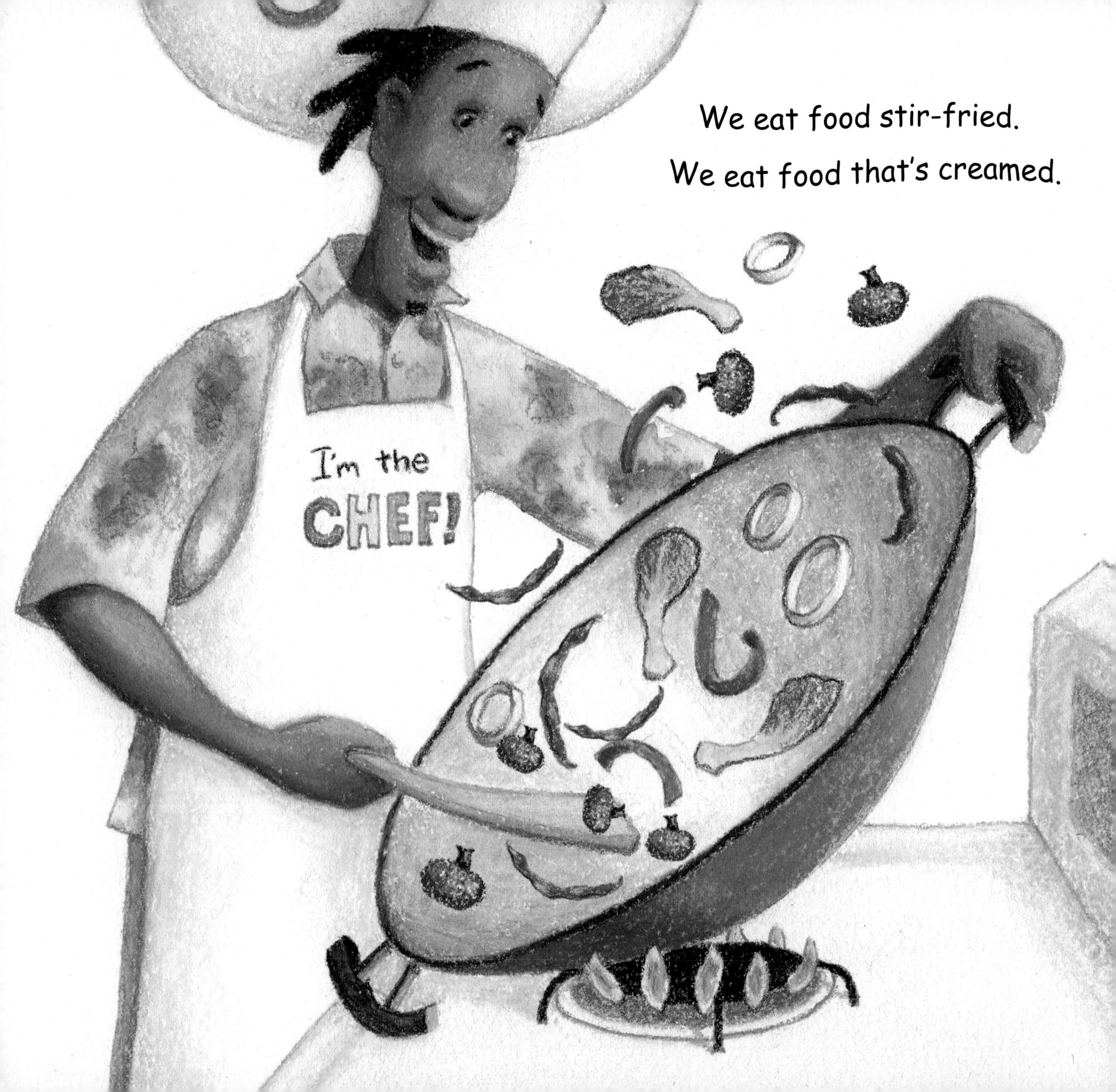

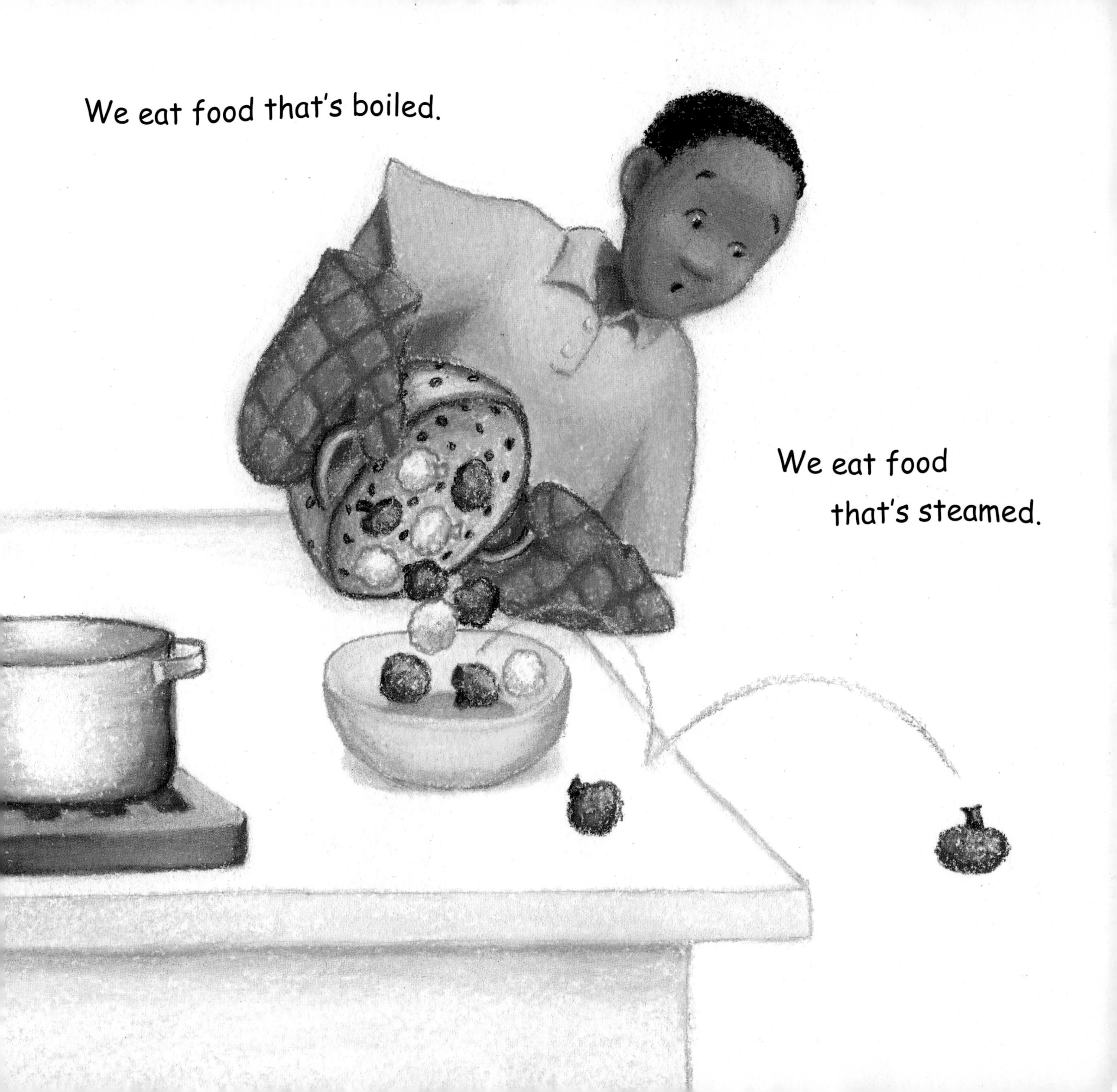

We eat food that's boiled.

We eat food
that's steamed.

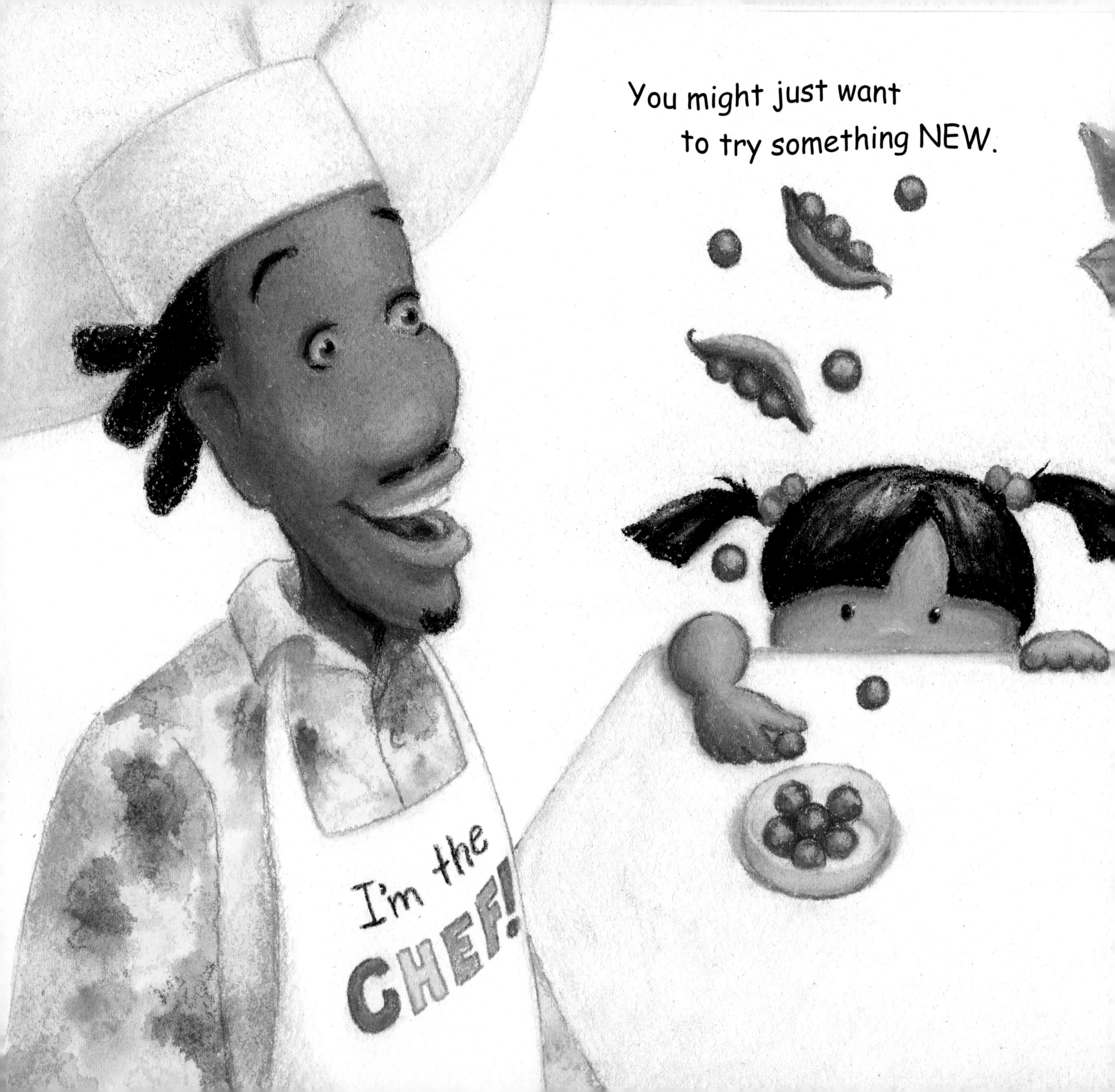

You might just want
to try something NEW.

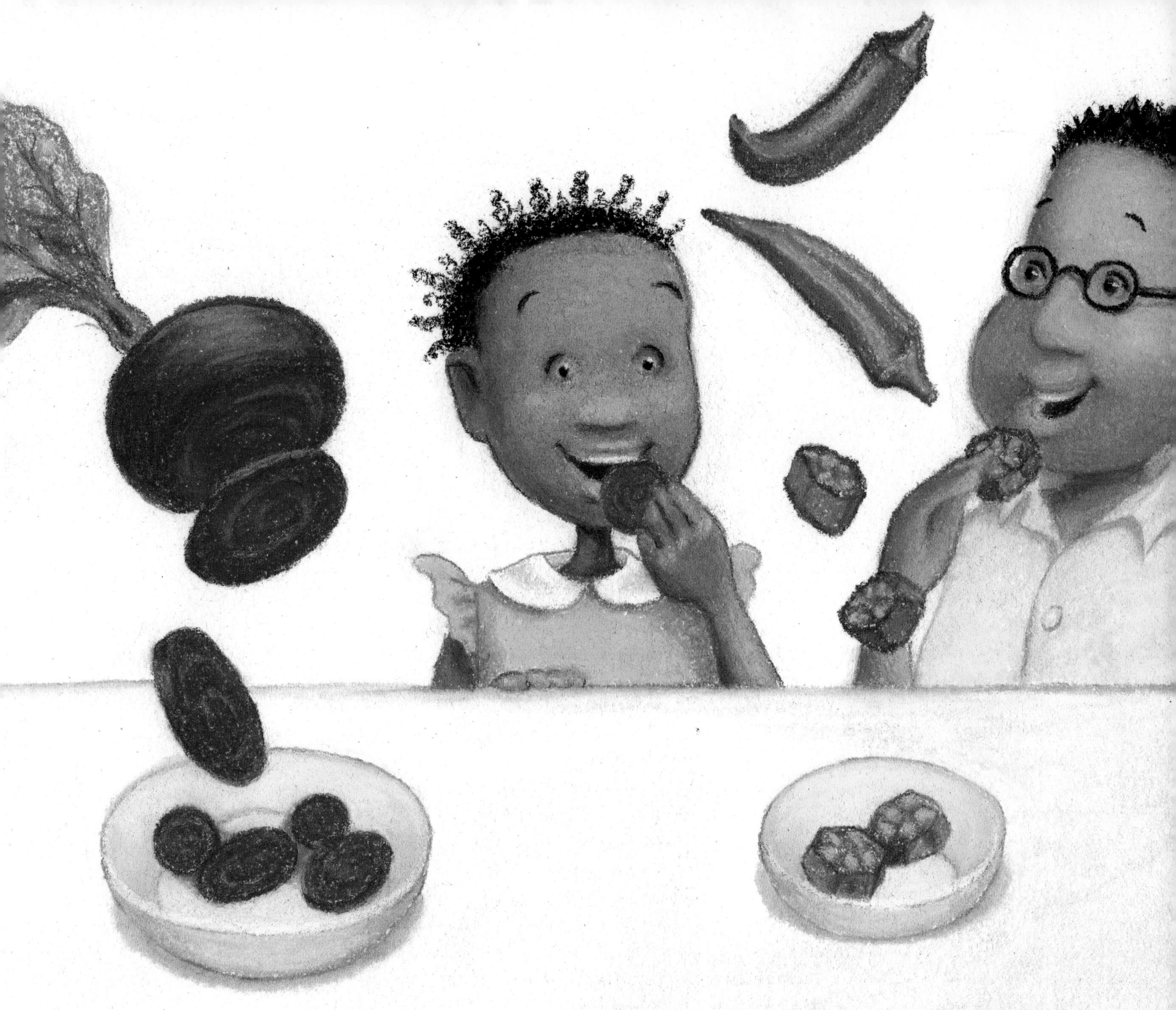

PEAS, BEETS, OKRA... are great veggies for you.

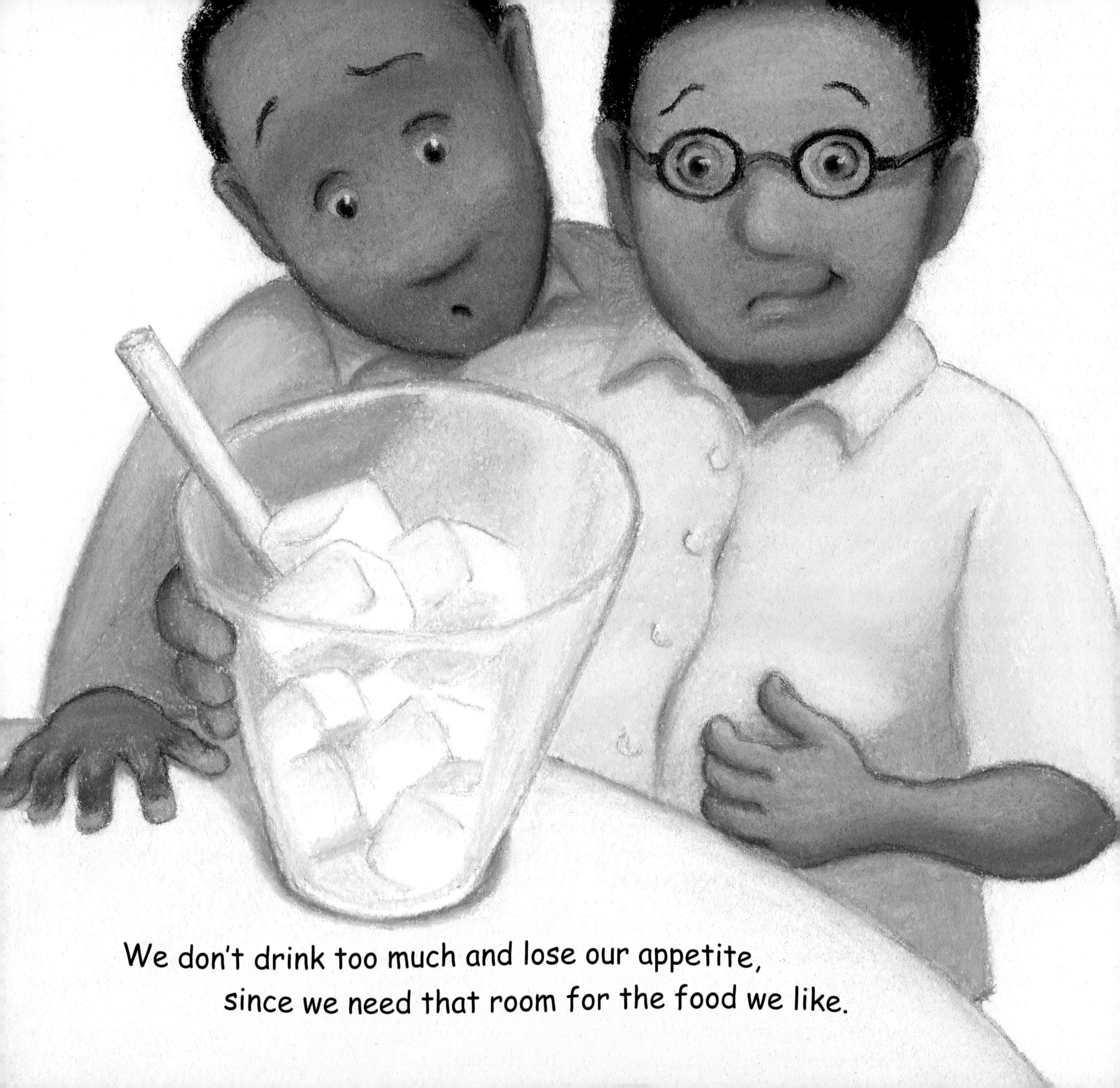

We don't drink too much and lose our appetite,
since we need that room for the food we like.

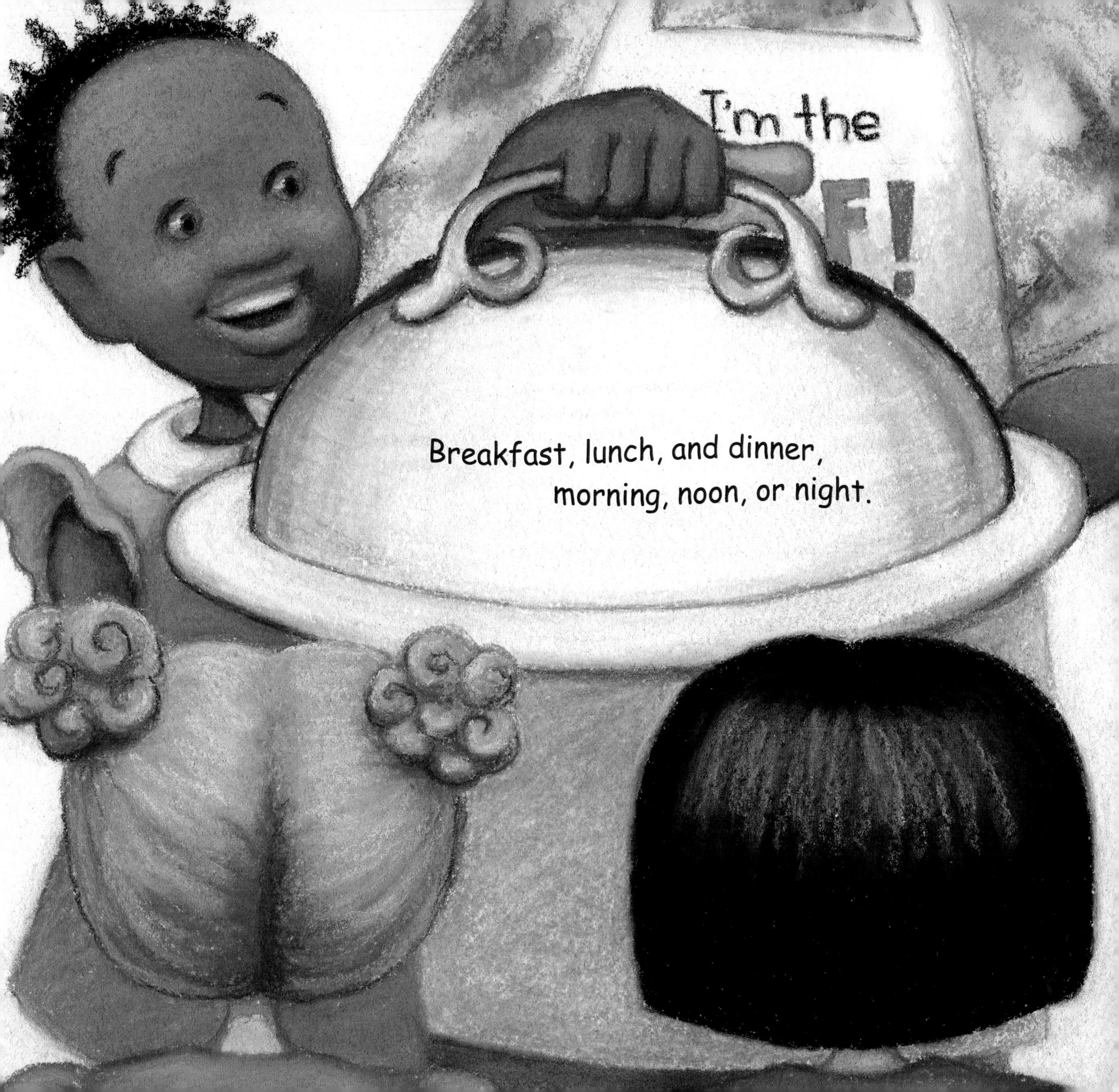

Breakfast, lunch, and dinner,
morning, noon, or night.

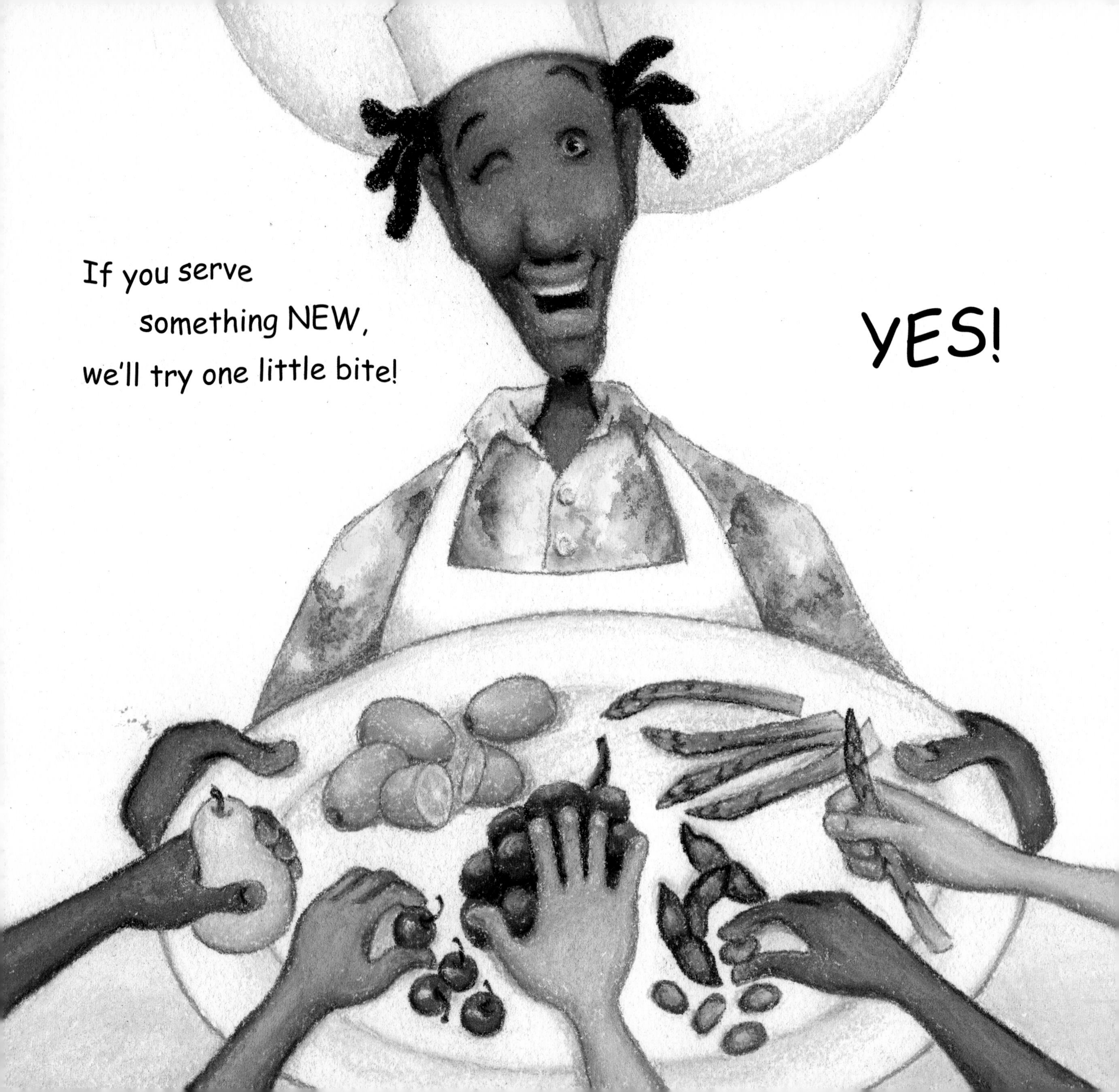
If you serve
something NEW,
we'll try one little bite!
YES!